ACID REFLUX
DIET COOKBOOK

Manage GERD & LPR, Improve Digestion, and Enjoy a Life Free from
Discomfort with Tasty, Nutrient-Rich Recipes | Includes Expert
Advice & a Heartburn-Free 60-Day Meal Plan

Nicòle Everglen

TABLE OF CONTENTS

INTRODUCTION

"Health is not valued till sickness comes."
– Thomas Fuller

"The modern life has birthed an array of health issues," is a cliché we've heard often, but it's true. The present lifestyles we live are significantly altering the well-being of individuals across the globe. Sedentary behaviors, poor dietary habits, high stress levels, and an overreliance on processed foods have all contributed to a surge in lifestyle-related diseases. The relentless pursuit of convenience and immediate gratification has led to neglecting the foundational principles of health, manifesting in conditions such as obesity, diabetes, cardiovascular diseases, and, notably, gastrointestinal disorders.

Among these ailments, the US population stands particularly at risk. The prevalence of fast food, combined with a culture that prioritizes work over wellness, exacerbates our vulnerability. The American diet, often high in fats, sugars, and processed ingredients, is largely to blame. Coupled with a tendency towards larger portion sizes and irregular meal patterns, our culinary industry has created a breeding ground for various health complications. The enemy we're dealing with in this book is acid reflux.

Acid reflux, also known as gastroesophageal reflux disease (GERD), is a condition where stomach acid frequently flows back into the esophagus, causing irritation and discomfort. This disease affects a significant portion of the US population, with studies estimating that nearly 20% of Americans experience symptoms of GERD on a weekly basis. These symptoms, which include heartburn, regurgitation, and chest pain, can severely impact the quality of life if left unmanaged. The need for effective and sustainable solutions to manage and alleviate acid reflux has never been more critical.

The *Acid Reflux Diet Cookbook* was written for one purpose: to provide you with a comprehensive understanding of acid reflux, its causes, and effective ways to manage it through diet and lifestyle changes. The first part of the book delves into the science of acid reflux, offering detailed, science-based explanations of how and why the condition occurs. Following this, we will explore food items specifically designed for managing acid reflux. You will learn about the foods to avoid and those that can help alleviate symptoms. The final section of the book features a collection of 70 carefully curated recipes that are both delicious and beneficial for those suffering from acid reflux. From breakfast to dinner, snacks to desserts, these recipes are designed to minimize symptoms while ensuring you do not have to compromise on taste or variety. Each recipe comes with detailed nutritional information, making it easy for you to monitor your intake and maintain a balanced diet.

As a resident of the United States, you might find this book particularly beneficial due to its targeted approach to the unique challenges faced by the American people.

It doesn't matter if you are newly diagnosed with acid reflux or have been managing it for a while, by the end of this book, we hope to make your life easier through informed dietary choices.

Chapter 1

THE SCIENCE OF ACID REFLUX

We can't make informed choices if we are ignorant of the facts. Let's start with uncovering the science of this disease. Acid reflux occurs when the contents of the stomach, including gastric acid, flow back into the esophagus, the tube that connects the throat to the stomach. This backflow, or reflux, is primarily caused by the malfunction of the lower esophageal sphincter (LES), a ring-like muscle that acts as a valve between the esophagus and the stomach. Under normal circumstances, the LES opens to allow food to enter the stomach and closes to prevent stomach contents from flowing back into the esophagus. However, when the LES is weak or relaxes inappropriately, stomach acid can escape into the esophagus, leading to acid reflux.

The LES is a critical structure in the gastrointestinal tract, situated at the junction of the esophagus and the stomach. It is composed of smooth muscle fibers that maintain tonic contraction to prevent reflux. Upon swallowing, the LES transiently relaxes to allow the passage of food into the stomach, then contracts again to seal off the esophagus from the stomach contents. This precise coordination is what maintains the barrier between the stomach and the esophagus. When the LES fails to close properly or opens too frequently, the acidic contents of the stomach can flow back into the esophagus. This reflux of acid irritates the esophageal lining, which is not equipped to handle such acidity, unlike the stomach lining which has protective mechanisms. The repeated exposure of the esophagus to stomach acid can lead to inflammation and damage, a condition known as esophagitis.

The esophagus has its own defense mechanisms to combat occasional reflux. These include peristalsis, a coordinated muscular contraction that helps clear the esophagus of its contents, and the production of saliva, which contains bicarbonate to neutralize acid. However, these mechanisms can be overwhelmed by frequent and severe reflux, leading to chronic symptoms and complications. This knowledge is crucial for devising effective strategies for managing and treating acid reflux, which we will explore further in the subsequent sections of this book.

DIFFERENCES BETWEEN GERD AND LPR

"Acid Reflux" itself can be confused for two separate conditions. While GERD (Gastroesophageal Reflux Disease) and LPR (Laryngopharyngeal Reflux) both involve the reflux of stomach contents, they differ significantly in affected areas, symptoms, and underlying mechanisms. The issue we are tackling is GERD, and when we say Acid Reflux, this is the condition we're referring to. The following information will help you discern if you're experiencing GERD or LPR.

Affected Areas

GERD primarily affects the esophagus. This occurs due to the malfunction of the lower esophageal sphincter (LES), which is the muscle at the junction of the esophagus and stomach. When the LES fails to close properly, stomach acid flows back into the esophagus, causing irritation and inflammation.

LPR affects the larynx (voice box) and pharynx (throat). It involves the upper esophageal sphincter (UES), which is the muscle at the junction of the esophagus and throat. LPR allows stomach acid to reach the upper airway and throat, leading to irritation and inflammation in those areas.

Symptoms

GERD presents with symptoms such as heartburn, regurgitation, chest pain, difficulty swallowing, chronic cough, and hoarseness. The most common and distinctive symptom is heartburn, a burning sensation in the chest.

LPR, on the other hand, often presents without the typical heartburn. Its symptoms include chronic cough, hoarseness, sore throat, a sensation of a lump in the throat, difficulty swallowing, postnasal drip, and frequent throat clearing. Due to the lack of heartburn, LPR is often referred to as "silent reflux."

Mechanisms

In GERD, the LES dysfunction allows stomach acid to flow back into the esophagus. This reflux leads to inflammation and damage to the esophageal lining. Factors such as obesity, certain foods, smoking, and medications can contribute to LES dysfunction and GERD.

LPR occurs when the UES fails to prevent stomach acid from reaching the larynx and pharynx. This reflux causes irritation and inflammation in the upper airway and throat. LPR can be triggered by dietary factors, stress, and medical conditions like asthma and sinusitis. It involves both LES and UES dysfunction.

Common Causes

GERD is commonly caused by obesity, hiatal hernia, pregnancy, smoking, certain medications (e.g., NSAIDs, some blood pressure medications), and dietary factors such as fatty foods, chocolate, caffeine, and alcohol.

LPR shares similar causes but places more emphasis on the dysfunction of both the LES and UES. Dietary factors, stress, and certain medical conditions can also contribute to LPR.

Understanding these distinctions helps tailor the management strategies for GERD and LPR, ensuring effective and appropriate treatment based on their unique presentations and underlying causes.

SYMPTOMS AND CAUSES OF ACID REFLUX

Symptoms of Acid Reflux

1. **Heartburn**: A burning sensation in the chest, often after eating, which might be worse at night or when lying down.
2. **Regurgitation**: A sour or bitter-tasting acid backing up into your throat or mouth.
3. **Chest Pain**: Discomfort or pain in the chest, especially after eating or lying down.
4. **Difficulty Swallowing (Dysphagia)**: A sensation of food being stuck in the throat.
5. **Chronic Cough**: A persistent cough that does not seem to be related to respiratory conditions.
6. **Hoarseness or Sore Throat**: A raspy voice or a persistent sore throat.
7. **Sensation of a Lump in the Throat**: Feeling like there's a lump in your throat that doesn't go away.
8. **Bloating and Burping**: Frequent burping and bloating, especially after meals.

Causes of Acid Reflux

1. **Lower Esophageal Sphincter (LES) Dysfunction**: The LES should close as soon as food passes through it. If it doesn't close all the way or if it opens too often, acid produced by your stomach can move up into your esophagus, causing acid reflux.
2. **Hiatal Hernia**: This occurs when the upper part of the stomach moves up into the chest through a small opening in the diaphragm, making it easier for acid to move up into the esophagus. Hiatal hernias are common and the risk increases with age.
3. **Obesity**: Excess weight can put pressure on the abdomen, pushing up the stomach and causing acid to back up into the esophagus. Individuals with a body mass index (BMI) over 30 are at a higher risk of experiencing acid reflux.
4. **Pregnancy**: Increased levels of hormones during pregnancy can relax the LES, while the growing fetus can put pressure on the stomach. Acid reflux is common during the second and third trimesters of pregnancy.
5. **Diet**: Certain foods and drinks, including fatty or fried foods, chocolate, caffeine, alcohol, spicy foods, garlic, onions, and acidic foods like citrus fruits and tomatoes, can trigger acid reflux.
6. **Smoking**: Smoking can impair muscle reflexes in the throat and increase acid production. Smokers are more likely to develop GERD compared to non-smokers.
7. **Medications**: Certain medications, such as aspirin, ibuprofen, certain muscle relaxers, or blood pressure medications, can cause acid reflux.
8. **Lying Down After Eating**: Lying down or going to bed shortly after eating can promote acid reflux. It is recommended to wait at least 2-3 hours after eating before lying down.
9. **Eating Large Meals**: Consuming large meals can increase abdominal pressure and promote reflux. Smaller, more frequent meals are often advised to help mitigate symptoms.

CORRELATION BETWEEN GERD, HIATAL HERNIA AND THE VAGUS NERVE

GERD (Gastroesophageal Reflux Disease), hiatal hernia, and the **vagus nerve** are interconnected conditions through their roles in the digestive system and their impact on the lower esophageal sphincter (LES) function. If you're suffering from one, chances are you are suffering from the other, or are at least susceptible to it. A hiatal hernia occurs when part of the stomach pushes up through the diaphragm into the chest cavity. There are two main types:

- **Sliding Hiatal Hernia**: The more common type, where the stomach and the section of the esophagus that joins the stomach slide up into the chest through the hiatus.
- **Paraesophageal Hiatal Hernia**: Less common but more serious, where part of the stomach pushes through the hiatus and sits next to the esophagus.

This condition is linked with GERD in several ways, namely:

1. **Disruption of LES Function**: The diaphragm normally helps the LES keep stomach acid from backing up into the esophagus. A hiatal hernia can disrupt this function, weakening the LES and allowing acid reflux.
2. **Increased Intra-Abdominal Pressure**: Hiatal hernias can increase pressure on the stomach, promoting the backflow of stomach contents into the esophagus.
3. **Anatomical Changes**: The anatomical displacement caused by a hiatal hernia can alter the angle at which the esophagus enters the stomach, making it easier for acid to reflux.

What about the vagus nerve? It's a critical component of the autonomic nervous system, controlling parasympathetic functions. It extends from the brainstem through the neck and thorax down to the abdomen, innervating multiple organs, including the heart, lungs, and digestive tract. It affects GERD through the following factors:

1. **Regulation of LES Tone**: The vagus nerve controls the tone and relaxation of the LES. Proper signaling helps maintain the LES's ability to close tightly after food passes into the stomach, preventing reflux.

2. **Gastric Motility**: The vagus nerve regulates stomach acid production and gastric emptying. Dysfunctional vagus nerve signaling can lead to delayed gastric emptying, increasing the risk of reflux as food and acid linger longer in the stomach.

3. **Esophageal Peristalsis**: The vagus nerve also influences esophageal peristalsis, the wave-like muscle contractions that move food down the esophagus. Impaired peristalsis can lead to incomplete clearance of refluxed acid, exacerbating GERD symptoms.

To summarize their link, a hiatal hernia can physically interfere with the vagus nerve, potentially disrupting its signaling pathways, which in turn triggers reflexive responses that complicate LES control and gastric functions.

CONNECTION BETWEEN ACID REFLUX AND COUGH

Have you been experiencing unrelenting cough but no cold? Acid reflux may be the reason. The two are closely related due to the irritation caused by stomach acid when it refluxes into the esophagus and sometimes even into the throat and larynx. This may be misconstrued as LPR, but the cause for this is GERD as the origin point of the condition is different. This backflow of acid can stimulate the nerve endings in these areas, leading to a chronic cough. When acid escapes the stomach and irritates the lining of the esophagus, it can trigger a cough reflex as the body attempts to clear the irritating substance from the esophageal lining.

Additionally, acid reflux can cause micro-aspirations, where small amounts of stomach acid reach the upper respiratory tract, including the larynx and the lungs. This can cause inflammation and irritation in these areas, leading to coughing. The frequent exposure to acid can also damage the tissues in the throat, leading to chronic inflammation and a persistent cough. This is particularly common in Laryngopharyngeal Reflux (LPR), the silent reflux, where people may not experience the typical heartburn symptoms but suffer from respiratory symptoms like coughing.

Moreover, GERD can exacerbate existing respiratory conditions such as asthma, leading to increased coughing. The presence of stomach acid in the esophagus can cause bronchoconstriction and increased mucus production, which are common in asthma patients. We explore this relationship in the next section.

LINK BETWEEN ACID REFLUX AND ASTHMA

Acid reflux and asthma are interconnected through several physiological mechanisms that exacerbate each condition. When stomach acid flows back into the esophagus, it can trigger a nerve reflex that causes the airways to constrict to prevent the acid from entering the lungs. This bronchoconstriction can lead to asthma symptoms such as wheezing, coughing, and shortness of breath.

If that isn't worrisome enough, the refluxed acid can also cause inflammation and swelling in the airways, further aggravating asthma. When acid reaches the throat and the upper airway, it can lead to LPR, which may not only cause throat irritation and coughing but can also trigger asthma symptoms by inflaming the respiratory tract. The chronic irritation and inflammation can make the airways more sensitive and reactive to asthma triggers.

Additionally, people with asthma are more likely to experience GERD. Asthma medications, particularly beta-agonists and theophylline, can relax the LES, making it easier for stomach acid to reflux into the esophagus. The frequent coughing associated with asthma can also increase abdominal pressure, promoting acid reflux. This bidirectional relationship creates a cycle where each condition exacerbates the other, making effective management crucial for patients suffering from both asthma and GERD—enforcing us to study our existing lifestyle closely and perform the necessary reforms to bring everything in line, particularly our diets.

THE FOUR STAGES OF GERD

GERD (Gastroesophageal Reflux Disease) progresses through four stages, each with increasing severity and associated complications.

Stage 1: Mild GERD

In the initial stage, patients experience occasional acid reflux, typically less than twice a week. Symptoms include mild heartburn and regurgitation, usually triggered by certain foods, stress, or lifestyle factors. This stage is common among younger adults who have recently developed poor dietary habits or increased stress levels. Overweight individuals are also at higher risk due to increased abdominal pressure, which promotes reflux. To manage this stage, we have to identify and avoid triggers by adopting a healthier diet, and making lifestyle changes such as losing weight, quitting smoking, and elevating the head during sleep.

Stage 2: Moderate GERD

During stage 2, the frequency of acid reflux episodes increases to several times a week. Symptoms become more persistent and severe, including frequent heartburn, regurgitation, and difficulty swallowing. This stage is prevalent among middle-aged adults who may have had GERD symptoms for several years. Pregnant women are also at higher risk during this stage due to hormonal changes and increased abdominal pressure from the growing fetus. At this stage, prescription medications such as proton pump inhibitors (PPIs) or H2 blockers are often required to manage symptoms and reduce acid production. Lifestyle changes continue to play an essential role in symptom management.

Stage 3: Severe GERD

Stage 3 is characterized by chronic and severe symptoms that occur daily. The esophagus shows signs of inflammation (esophagitis) and possible damage due to constant exposure to stomach acid. Populations at higher risk for this stage include older adults, especially those with a long history of untreated or poorly managed GERD. Individuals with hiatal hernia are also at significant risk, as the anatomical displacement exacerbates reflux. Complications such as esophageal strictures (narrowing of the esophagus due to scar tissue) and Barrett's esophagus (a precancerous condition where the esophageal lining changes) may develop. At this stage, patients typically require long-term medication management with PPIs, and more aggressive treatments may be considered. Regular monitoring by a healthcare professional is crucial to manage and mitigate complications.

Stage 4: Complicated GERD

In the final stage, GERD leads to significant complications and chronic symptoms that severely impact the patient's quality of life. Populations most at risk include older adults with a long-standing history of severe GERD, individuals with Barrett's esophagus, and those with other predisposing conditions such as obesity, smoking, and poor dietary habits. Barrett's esophagus and esophageal cancer are potential risks, and patients may suffer from severe esophagitis, significant esophageal strictures, and ulcers. Surgical intervention, such as fundoplication, may be recommended when medications and lifestyle changes are insufficient to control symptoms and prevent further damage. Endoscopic therapies may also be considered to manage Barrett's esophagus and prevent progression to cancer.

SHOULD YOU CONSIDER MEDICAL CONSULTATION?

If you find yourself experiencing heartburn more than twice a week, it's a strong indicator that your condition may be progressing beyond occasional discomfort. Persistent heartburn can signify chronic GERD, and a sign you should see a healthcare professional to prevent potential complications.

Are you noticing your symptoms getting worse despite over-the-counter treatments? It's time to seek medical advice. When medications like antacids or H2 blockers no longer provide relief, it suggests that the underlying issue might be more severe and requires professional evaluation.

Experiencing difficulty swallowing or feeling like food is getting stuck in your throat is another red flag. This can indicate esophageal damage or strictures, which need medical attention to prevent further complications.

Unexplained weight loss, persistent vomiting, or signs of gastrointestinal bleeding such as black or bloody stools, are also indicators that you should seek immediate medical care. These symptoms can signal severe complications from GERD, including esophagitis, ulcers, or even esophageal cancer.

Furthermore, if your acid reflux is disrupting your sleep or significantly affecting your quality of life, it's important to talk to a doctor. Chronic sleep disruption and continuous discomfort can lead to other health issues, and managing your GERD effectively can help improve your overall well-being.

Lastly, if you have a history of GERD and start experiencing new or worsening symptoms, it's a good idea to consult your doctor. Conditions like Barrett's esophagus, which is a precancerous state, need regular monitoring and management to prevent progression to esophageal cancer.

Your health and comfort are paramount, and addressing these symptoms with your healthcare provider can help you manage and treat acid reflux effectively, ensuring you maintain a good quality of life.

When Is Surgery Recommended?

Surgery is typically recommended for acid reflux, or GERD, in the following situations:

1. **Severe Symptoms Unresponsive to Medication**: If you have chronic and severe GERD symptoms that do not improve with medications such as proton pump inhibitors (PPIs) or H2 blockers, your doctor might suggest surgery.
2. **Complications from GERD**: When GERD leads to serious complications like severe esophagitis (inflammation of the esophagus), Barrett's esophagus (a precancerous condition), or esophageal strictures (narrowing of the esophagus), surgical intervention may be necessary.
3. **Intolerance to Medications**: If you experience significant side effects from GERD medications or prefer not to take them long-term, surgery might be considered.
4. **Hiatal Hernia**: If a hiatal hernia is contributing to your GERD symptoms, repairing the hernia through surgery can be beneficial.

Types of Surgery for GERD

1. **Nissen Fundoplication**: This is the most common surgical procedure for GERD. The surgeon wraps the top of the stomach around the lower esophagus to strengthen the LES, preventing acid reflux.
2. **Laparoscopic Surgery**: A minimally invasive approach where small incisions are made in the abdomen to perform the surgery using a laparoscope (a small camera).
3. **LINX Device**: A ring of magnetic beads is placed around the LES to reinforce it and prevent acid reflux while allowing food to pass through.
4. **Endoscopic Procedures**: Less invasive techniques such as the TIF (Transoral Incisionless Fundoplication) procedure, where the LES is repaired using an endoscope inserted through the mouth.

Surgical procedures can be terrifying, with complications haunting every surgeon's table. It's understandable if you don't want to opt for this route. That's why we are advocating for our a diet restructuring because when it comes to managing acid reflux, focusing on diet and lifestyle changes can be both effective and affordable. Let's explore some practical strategies that can help you alleviate symptoms and improve your quality of life.

Dietary Changes

Start by identifying and eliminating foods that trigger your acid reflux. Common culprits include fatty and fried foods, chocolate, caffeine, alcohol, spicy foods, garlic, onions, and acidic foods like citrus fruits and tomatoes. For a better understanding of prohibited foods, you may refer to Chapter 2.

Eating smaller, more frequent meals can also make a significant difference. Large meals can increase stomach pressure and promote reflux, so try to eat five to six smaller meals throughout the day instead of three large ones. This approach helps reduce stomach distension and minimizes reflux episodes.

Incorporating more alkaline foods into your diet can help neutralize stomach acid. Consider adding vegetables, melons, bananas, oatmeal, and ginger to your meals. These foods not only soothe the digestive tract but also reduce acid reflux symptoms. Staying hydrated is equally important; drink plenty of water throughout the day and avoid beverages that can trigger reflux, such as coffee, tea, and carbonated drinks.

Lifestyle Modifications

Excess weight can put pressure on your stomach, causing acid to back up into your esophagus. Achieving and maintaining a healthy weight through a balanced diet and regular exercise can significantly reduce acid reflux symptoms. Elevating the head of your bed by 6-8 inches can prevent acid from flowing back into the esophagus while you sleep. You can achieve this by using bed risers, wedge pillows, or an adjustable bed. Additionally, avoid lying down or going to bed immediately after eating. Wait at least 2-3 hours to allow your stomach to empty and reduce the risk of reflux. Wearing loose-fitting clothing can also help. Tight clothing, especially around the abdomen, can put pressure on your stomach and exacerbate acid reflux. Choose comfortable, loose-fitting clothes to alleviate this pressure.

Behavioral Changes

Chew your food thoroughly and eat slowly. Taking time to chew your food and eat at a slower pace aids in digestion and reduces the likelihood of acid reflux. Mindful eating can help you recognize when you are full and prevent overeating, which can also trigger reflux.

Managing stress is another vital aspect. Stress can exacerbate acid reflux symptoms, so incorporating stress-reducing techniques like deep breathing exercises, meditation, yoga, and regular physical activity can be beneficial. These practices help lower stress levels and, in turn, reduce reflux symptoms.

With thorough implementation of these changes, it's possible to successfully manage acid reflux. Let's get you started with the first step, dietary reform, in the upcoming chapters.

Chapter 2
DIET AND NUTRITION

I n the first chapter, we established science of acid reflux. How about going back to where it begins? The origin of acid reflux can often be traced back to a person's habits and lifestyle choices, which significantly impact the likelihood of experiencing this uncomfortable condition. Acid reflux, as we've understood, occurs when stomach acid flows back into the esophagus, causing symptoms such as heartburn, regurgitation, and discomfort. Several lifestyle factors contribute to this backward flow of acid, with diet and nutrition playing a central role.

Upon closer inspection, we can see how your dietary habits might be solely responsible. For the average American, smaller meals are rare. Consuming large meals can increase stomach pressure, which in turn forces the lower esophageal sphincter (LES) to open and allows acid to escape into the esophagus. Eating too quickly can also exacerbate this problem, as it leads to swallowing air and increases the volume in the stomach, contributing to reflux. Furthermore, the timing of meals is crucial; eating right before bedtime can worsen acid reflux because lying down makes it easier for stomach acid to flow back into the esophagus.

The types of foods and beverages consumed are equally important. High-fat foods, for instance, slow down stomach emptying, increasing the likelihood of reflux. Spicy foods, citrus fruits, chocolate, caffeine, and alcohol are also common triggers. These items can irritate the esophageal lining or relax the LES, allowing acid to escape. Carbonated drinks can cause bloating and put extra pressure on the LES, while acidic foods like tomatoes and vinegar can directly irritate the esophagus. We'll take a closer look at the list of allowed and prohibited foods later in this chapter.

Narrowing the focus to diet and nutrition, it becomes clear that making strategic changes in this area can significantly reduce acid reflux symptoms. If a diet with high triggers is the problem, then a diet with low to no triggers can be the solution; by adopting a diet that avoids known triggers and includes foods that support digestive health, you can manage your symptoms more effectively.

To divulge a bit more on the nature of diet and nutrition, the two encompass the selection and consumption of foods and beverages, along with their impact on the body's overall health and functioning. Nutrition involves understanding the nutrients in various foods and how they affect bodily processes, while diet refers to the patterns and types of foods consumed regularly. These two elements are foundational to maintaining health, preventing chronic diseases, and promoting longevity.

Proper nutrition provides the body with essential nutrients—such as vitamins, minerals, proteins, fats, and carbohydrates—that are crucial for maintaining bodily functions. Nutrients play a vital role in energy production, immune function, cell repair, and overall growth and development. A balanced diet ensures that the body receives these nutrients in adequate amounts to support optimal health. Conversely, poor dietary choices can lead to nutrient deficiencies, weakening the body's defense mechanisms and increasing susceptibility to illnesses like acid reflux.

But, wait; there's more. The significance of diet and nutrition extends beyond mere survival. They are pivotal in preserving health and enhancing quality of life. Consuming a variety of nutrient-dense foods helps in maintaining a healthy weight, reducing the risk of chronic diseases like heart disease, diabetes, and certain cancers, and promoting mental well-being. Foods rich in antioxidants, for example, help combat oxidative stress and inflammation, which are underlying factors in acid reflux. Hence, a well-balanced diet of acid-friendly foods contributes not only to immediate health benefits but also to long-term vitality and longevity.

Certain foods can either trigger or alleviate acid reflux symptoms. By understanding which foods to avoid and which to include, you can reduce the frequency and severity of acid reflux episodes. The prohibited foods listed are known to relax the lower esophageal sphincter (LES), increase stomach acid production, or irritate the esophagus, all of which can worsen acid reflux symptoms. Conversely, the allowed foods are typically low in acid, fat, and caffeine, and high in fiber and water content, which help neutralize stomach acid and promote healthy digestion. This guide aims to provide clear and actionable dietary recommendations to help you manage acid reflux effectively, improving your overall digestive health and quality of life.

DIFFERENT ACID REFLUX DIETS

1. Low-Acid Diet

A low-acid diet focuses on reducing the intake of acidic foods and beverages that can irritate the esophagus and increase stomach acid production. This diet helps by minimizing the direct contact of acidic substances with the esophagus, thus reducing symptoms such as heartburn and regurgitation.

- **Allowed Foods**: Non-citrus fruits (bananas, melons), vegetables (broccoli, green beans), lean proteins (chicken, turkey), whole grains (brown rice, oatmeal), and non-fat dairy products.
- **Avoided Foods**: Citrus fruits (oranges, lemons), tomatoes, onions, garlic, caffeinated beverages, alcohol, chocolate, and spicy foods.

2. Mediterranean Diet

The Mediterranean diet emphasizes whole, minimally processed foods and healthy fats, which can help reduce inflammation and promote digestive health. This diet's emphasis on fruits, vegetables, whole grains, and lean proteins provides a balanced approach that supports overall well-being and reduces the likelihood of acid reflux.

- **Allowed Foods**: Fresh fruits and vegetables, whole grains, nuts and seeds, legumes, lean proteins (fish, poultry), and healthy fats (olive oil).
- **Avoided Foods**: Red meat, processed foods, refined sugars, and high-fat dairy products.

3. GERD Diet

The GERD (Gastroesophageal Reflux Disease) diet is specifically designed to manage the symptoms of acid reflux by avoiding known triggers and including foods that are less likely to cause reflux. This diet helps by reducing the frequency and severity of reflux episodes.

- **Allowed Foods**: Whole grains, lean meats, low-fat dairy, and vegetables.
- **Avoided Foods**: High-fat foods, spicy foods, caffeine, alcohol, and carbonated beverages.

4. Plant-Based Diet

A plant-based diet focuses on consuming primarily plant-derived foods, which are generally lower in fat and less acidic. This diet can help manage acid reflux by providing a high intake of fiber, vitamins, and antioxidants, which support digestive health.

- **Allowed Foods**: Fruits, vegetables, legumes, nuts, seeds, and whole grains.
- **Avoided Foods**: Animal products, processed foods, refined grains, and sugars.

5. Anti-Inflammatory Diet

An anti-inflammatory diet aims to reduce inflammation in the body, which can help alleviate acid reflux symptoms. Foods rich in antioxidants and anti-inflammatory compounds can help soothe the digestive tract and reduce irritation.

- **Allowed Foods**: Fruits (berries, cherries), vegetables (leafy greens, broccoli), healthy fats (olive oil, avocado), lean proteins, and whole grains.
- **Avoided Foods**: Processed foods, red meat, refined sugars, and trans fats.

6. FODMAP Diet

The FODMAP diet reduces the intake of certain carbohydrates that can ferment in the gut and cause bloating, gas, and reflux symptoms. By avoiding high-FODMAP foods, individuals can reduce the pressure on the LES and minimize reflux.

- **Allowed Foods**: Low-FODMAP foods such as bananas, carrots, chicken, eggs, and oats.
- **Avoided Foods**: High-FODMAP foods like apples, garlic, onions, beans, and wheat.

7. DASH Diet

The DASH (Dietary Approaches to Stop Hypertension) diet is rich in fruits, vegetables, and low-fat dairy, which can also help manage acid reflux by promoting a healthy digestive system and reducing the intake of trigger foods.

- **Allowed Foods**: Fruits, vegetables, whole grains, low-fat dairy, and lean proteins.
- **Avoided Foods**: High-fat, sugary, and salty foods.

8. Elimination Diet

An elimination diet involves removing potential trigger foods from your diet to identify which ones cause symptoms and then gradually reintroducing them. This personalized approach helps individuals pinpoint specific foods that trigger their acid reflux.

- **Allowed Foods**: Typically starts with safe foods like rice, turkey, and certain vegetables, then reintroduces other foods gradually.
- **Avoided Foods**: All suspected trigger foods initially, such as dairy, gluten, and caffeine.

9. Gluten-Free Diet

For those who are sensitive to gluten, following a gluten-free diet can help reduce acid reflux symptoms by eliminating foods that can cause inflammation and irritation in the digestive tract.

- **Allowed Foods**: Fruits, vegetables, gluten-free grains (quinoa, rice), lean proteins, and dairy substitutes.
- **Avoided Foods**: Wheat, barley, rye, and any products containing gluten.

Benefits of Each Diet for Acid Reflux

Each of these diets helps manage acid reflux by focusing on different aspects of food and nutrition:

- **Low-Acid and GERD Diets**: Directly reduce acid exposure and irritation in the esophagus.
- **Mediterranean and Anti-Inflammatory Diets**: Promote overall digestive health and reduce inflammation.
- **Plant-Based and DASH Diets**: Emphasize whole, minimally processed foods that support a healthy digestive system.
- **FODMAP and Elimination Diets**: Help identify and eliminate specific triggers for personalized management.
- **Gluten-Free Diet**: Reduces inflammation and irritation for those with gluten sensitivity.

We'll be taking a hybrid approach, not following any one diet's philosophy but carefully crafting recipes with a range of known acid-reducing and/or alkaline food items. If you're new to dieting as a whole, the next section might be worth a read.

MANAGING AN ACID REFLUX DIET

Imagine Sarah, a 35-year-old graphic designer who has been struggling with severe acid reflux for the past year. Her condition often disrupts her work and personal life, causing discomfort and anxiety about her meals. After a particularly bad episode, Sarah decides it's time to take control and systematically monitor her symptoms to identify triggers and manage her condition better. Here's how Sarah implements a comprehensive monitoring guide to help manage her acid reflux.

Keeping a Symptom Diary

Sarah starts by keeping a detailed symptom diary. Each day, she notes down the specific date and time of any reflux episodes, the symptoms she experiences, their duration, and their intensity.

Example Entry:

- **Date and Time**: June 20, 2024, 2:00 PM
- **Symptoms:** Burning sensation in the chest, mild nausea
- **Duration:** 30 minutes
- **Intensity**: 6/10

By doing this consistently, Sarah can track when her symptoms occur and how severe they are, which will help her identify patterns over time.

Tracking Food and Drink Intake

Sarah records everything she eats and drinks throughout the day, including portion sizes and specific ingredients, especially those known to trigger acid reflux.

Example Entry:

- **Time**: 1:00 PM
- **Meal:** Grilled chicken sandwich with lettuce, tomato, and mayonnaise; glass of water
- **Portion Size**: Whole sandwich, 8 oz water

This helps Sarah identify any correlation between her diet and her symptoms. She notices, for instance, that tomatoes often appear in her diary entries on days when her reflux is particularly bad.

Monitoring Lifestyle Factors

Sarah also tracks lifestyle factors such as physical activity, stress levels, sleep patterns, and any medications she takes.

Example Entry:

- **Activity**: Light exercise (walking) at 3:00 PM
- **Stress Level**: Moderate due to work deadlines
- **Sleep**: Went to bed at 10:30 PM, slept on left side
- **Medications**: Took 1 antacid tablet at 4:00 PM

By including this information, Sarah can see how non-dietary factors might be contributing to her reflux. For example, she realizes that stressful workdays often correlate with worse symptoms, indicating that stress management could be an important part of her treatment plan.

Identifying Patterns and Triggers

After a few weeks of diligent tracking, Sarah reviews her symptom diary and notices certain patterns. Spicy foods, tomatoes, and large meals late at night are common triggers. She also finds that her symptoms are worse on days when she's particularly stressed or eats quickly.

Sarah decides to eliminate these trigger foods from her diet, avoid eating large meals late at night, and practice stress management techniques such as meditation and deep breathing exercises.

Using Digital Tools and Apps

To make tracking easier, Sarah downloads a symptom tracking app. These apps often come with features like reminders, symptom tracking, and data visualization to help identify patterns more easily.

Recommended Apps:

- **MyFitnessPal**: For tracking food intake and exercise
- **Cara Care**: For managing gastrointestinal issues, including acid reflux
- **Symple Symptom Tracker**: For logging symptoms and potential triggers

Using these tools, Sarah can quickly input data and generate reports that provide a clear visual representation of her symptom patterns and potential triggers.

Consulting with Healthcare Providers

Sarah regularly shares her symptom diary with her healthcare provider. This helps her doctor understand her condition better and adjust her treatment plan as necessary.

What to Discuss:

- **Symptom Patterns**: Sarah and her doctor discuss any noticeable patterns or triggers.
- **Treatment Efficacy**: They review how well current treatments are managing her symptoms.
- **Adjustments**: They consider any necessary adjustments to diet, lifestyle, or medications.
  By maintaining open communication with her healthcare provider, Sarah ensures she receives personalized advice and treatment adjustments that cater to her specific needs.

Maintaining Consistency

Consistency is key for Sarah. She makes it a habit to log her symptoms, food intake, and lifestyle factors daily. This helps her gather comprehensive data that provides valuable insights into her condition.

To do this yourself, just place yourself in Sarah's shows and follow along each step. Keeping a detailed symptom diary, tracking food and lifestyle factors, using digital tools, and consulting with healthcare providers are all essential steps in this journey. This proactive approach will allow you to identify and manage triggers, leading to fewer symptoms and a healthier, more comfortable life.

FOODS TO AVOID

Now that you're familiar with the diet and nutrition aspect of managing acid reflux symptoms, we can start going to specific foods you should or shouldn't indulge in. The prohibited list for managing acid reflux contains many items that are staples in the American diet, such as tomatoes and tomato-based products, chocolate, caffeinated beverages, and fried foods. These foods are common in various popular dishes and beverages, including pizzas, pastas, sodas, and fast food. Additionally, items like high-fat dairy products, processed meats, and carbonated drinks are frequently consumed in typical American meals. The prevalence of these foods in everyday eating habits underscores a cultural challenge: how do you avoid something so widespread? The answer? Identify and eliminate.

1. **Alcohol**: Relaxes the LES and increases stomach acid production.
2. **Almond Milk (Sweetened and High-Fat Varieties)**: Certain varieties may trigger reflux due to added sugars and fat.
3. **Bacon**: High fat content can relax the LES and delay stomach emptying.

4. **Baked Goods (Brownies, Cakes)**: High fat and sugar content can delay stomach emptying and trigger reflux.
5. **Barbecue Sauce**: Often contains tomatoes, vinegar, and spices that can cause reflux.
6. **Buffalo Wings**: Combination of high fat and spicy sauce can exacerbate reflux symptoms.
7. **Butter and Cream**: High fat content can delay stomach emptying and relax the LES.
8. **Caffeinated Beverages (Coffee, Tea, Energy Drinks)**: Can relax the LES and increase stomach acid production.
9. **Carbonated Drinks**: Cause bloating and increase pressure on the LES, promoting reflux.
10. **Certain Nuts (Macadamia Nuts, Pecans)**: High fat content can trigger reflux symptoms.
11. **Certain Salad Dressings (Creamy or Acidic)**: High fat and acidic content can trigger reflux.
12. **Cheese (Especially High-Fat Varieties)**: High fat content can trigger reflux symptoms.
13. **Chili**: Combination of spicy ingredients and fatty meat can worsen reflux.
14. **Chocolate**: Contains caffeine and theobromine, which can relax the LES and increase acid reflux.
15. **Citrus Fruits (Oranges, Lemons, Grapefruits)**: High acidity can irritate the esophagus lining and exacerbate reflux symptoms.
16. **Citrus Juices**: Similar to citrus fruits, the high acidity can exacerbate reflux symptoms.
17. **Coconut Milk (Full-Fat)**: High fat content can delay stomach emptying and relax the LES.
18. **Corn Chips**: High fat and salt content can exacerbate reflux.
19. **Cream Cheese**: High fat content can relax the LES and delay stomach emptying.
20. **Cream-Based Soups**: High fat content can trigger reflux.
21. **Doughnuts and Pastries**: High fat and sugar content can delay stomach emptying and trigger reflux.
22. **French Fries**: High fat content can delay stomach emptying and trigger reflux.
23. **Fried Foods (Fried Chicken, etc.)**: High fat content slows stomach emptying, increasing the risk of acid reflux.
24. **Fudge and Caramel**: High sugar and fat content can delay stomach emptying and trigger reflux.
25. **Full-Fat Yogurt**: High fat content can relax the LES and delay stomach emptying.
26. **Garlic**: Can cause irritation and increase stomach acid production.
27. **Granola Bars with Chocolate or High-Fat Ingredients**: Can relax the LES and increase reflux.
28. **Granola with Added Sugars**: High sugar content can increase stomach acid production.
29. **Hamburgers**: High fat content, especially with added cheese and condiments, can promote reflux.
30. **High-Fat Dairy Products**: High fat content can relax the LES and delay stomach emptying.
31. **Hot Peppers**: High capsaicin content can irritate the esophagus and stomach lining.
32. **Ice Cream**: High fat and sugar content can trigger acid reflux.
33. **Ketchup**: Contain high levels of acid that can irritate the esophagus.
34. **Lasagna**: High fat and acidic tomato sauce can exacerbate reflux symptoms.
35. **Macaroni and Cheese**: High fat content can trigger reflux symptoms.
36. **Meatloaf**: High fat content can promote reflux symptoms.
37. **Mint (Peppermint, Mint-flavored Foods)**: Can relax the LES, allowing stomach acid to flow back into the esophagus.
38. **Mustard**: Contains vinegar and spices that can trigger reflux.
39. **Nachos with Cheese and Spicy Toppings**: High fat and spice content can exacerbate reflux.
40. **Onions (Raw and Cooked)**: Can cause belching and trigger acid reflux due to high acid content.
41. **Pancakes and Waffles (with Butter and Syrup)**: High fat and sugar content can promote reflux.
42. **Pasta with Tomato Sauce**: The tomato sauce's acidity can cause reflux symptoms.
43. **Pepper Jack Cheese**: Spicy and high-fat content can exacerbate reflux.
44. **Pepperoni**: High-fat content can relax the LES and promote reflux.

45. **Pickles and Pickled Vegetables**: High vinegar content makes them highly acidic.
46. **Pizza**: Combination of fatty cheese, acidic tomato sauce, and possibly spicy toppings can trigger reflux.
47. **Pork Chops (Fatty Cuts)**: High fat content can increase reflux risk.
48. **Potato Chips**: High fat and salt content can promote acid reflux.
49. **Processed Meats**: High fat content can relax the LES and increase reflux.
50. **Ribs and Other Fatty Meats**: High fat content can promote reflux.
51. **Salami**: High fat and spices can trigger reflux symptoms.
52. **Salsa**: Contains tomatoes and often spicy ingredients that can trigger reflux.
53. **Sausages**: High fat and spices can irritate the esophagus and promote reflux.
54. **Shortening and Lard**: High fat content can delay stomach emptying and promote reflux.
55. **Sour Candies**: High acidity can increase reflux symptoms.
56. **Spaghetti Bolognese**: Acidic tomato sauce and fatty meat can trigger reflux.
57. **Spicy Foods (Spicy Snacks, Salsa, Spicy Toppings)**: Can irritate the esophagus and increase stomach acid production, leading to reflux.
58. **Tomatoes and Tomato-Based Products**: High acidity can cause heartburn and worsen acid reflux.
59. **Vinegar**: Highly acidic and can irritate the esophagus lining.
60. **Whipped Cream**: High fat content can relax the LES and trigger reflux.

FOODS THAT HELP MANAGE ACID REFLUX

The allowed foods we have selected are common and can typically be found in major grocery chains such as Walmart, Kroger, Safeway, and Whole Foods. Specialty items like aloe vera, quinoa, chia seeds, and flax seeds might be found in the health food or organic sections.

1. **Acorn Squash**: Similar to butternut squash, it is low in acid and high in fiber.
2. **Almonds**: A good source of healthy fats that can help soothe the digestive tract.
3. **Aloe Vera**: Known for its soothing properties, it can help reduce inflammation in the stomach.
4. **Apples (Non-Citrus Varieties)**: Low in acid and can help reduce symptoms of acid reflux.
5. **Applesauce**: A low-acid fruit option that can be easy on the stomach.
6. **Artichokes**: Low in acid and high in fiber, beneficial for managing reflux.
7. **Asparagus**: Low in acid and can help reduce symptoms of reflux.
8. **Avocado**: Contains healthy fats that can help soothe the digestive tract.
9. **Bananas**: Low in acid and can help soothe the stomach.
10. **Barley**: High in fiber and can help reduce symptoms of reflux.
11. **Beets**: Low in acid and high in fiber, beneficial for managing reflux.
12. **Brussels Sprouts**: Low in acid and high in fiber, making them a good choice for managing reflux.
13. **Butternut Squash**: Low in acid and high in fiber, making it a good choice for managing reflux.
14. **Carrots**: Low in acid and high in fiber, making them a good choice for managing reflux.
15. **Cauliflower**: Low in acid and can be a soothing food option.
16. **Celery**: Low in calories and high in water content, it can help neutralize stomach acid.
17. **Chard**: Another green vegetable that is beneficial for managing reflux.
18. **Chia Seeds**: High in fiber and omega-3 fatty acids, which can help reduce inflammation.
19. **Chicken Broth (Low-Fat)**: A soothing and low-fat option that can be easy on the stomach.
20. **Chickpeas**: High in fiber and protein, which can help manage symptoms of reflux.
21. **Couscous**: A low-fat grain that can help manage reflux symptoms.
22. **Cucumber**: High in water content and low in acid, which can help neutralize stomach acid.
23. **Edamame**: High in fiber and protein, making it a good option for managing reflux.
24. **Egg Whites**: Low in fat and a good source of protein, avoiding the fatty yolk.

25. **Fennel**: Has natural soothing properties and can help improve digestion.
26. **Flax Seeds**: Another source of fiber and omega-3 fatty acids, beneficial for managing reflux.
27. **Ginger**: Known for its natural anti-inflammatory properties, it can help reduce gastric irritation and improve digestion.
28. **Greek Yogurt (Low-Fat)**: High in protein and can help improve digestion.
29. **Green Beans**: Low in acid and high in fiber, making them a good choice for reducing reflux.
30. **Green Peas**: Low in acid and high in fiber, beneficial for managing reflux.
31. **Green Vegetables (Broccoli, Spinach)**: Low in acid and high in fiber, they help maintain a healthy digestive system and can reduce symptoms of reflux.
32. **Herbal Teas (Chamomile, Licorice)**: Can soothe the digestive tract and reduce symptoms of acid reflux.
33. **Kale**: A green vegetable that is low in acid and high in fiber.
34. **Lean Meats (Chicken, Turkey)**: Low-fat proteins that are less likely to trigger reflux compared to fatty meats.
35. **Lentils**: Another high-fiber and protein-rich option that is easy on the stomach.
36. **Melons (Watermelon, Cantaloupe)**: Low in acid and high in water content, which can help neutralize stomach acid.
37. **Non-Citrus Fruits**: Low in acid, they are gentle on the stomach and can help soothe symptoms of acid reflux.
38. **Oatmeal**: A low-fat, high-fiber food that can absorb stomach acid and reduce symptoms of reflux.
39. **Oats**: High in fiber and can absorb stomach acid, reducing symptoms.
40. **Parsley**: Known for its soothing properties and can help improve digestion.
41. **Pears**: Another low-acid fruit that can be soothing to the digestive system.
42. **Polenta**: A low-fat, high-fiber food that can help manage symptoms of reflux.
43. **Popcorn (Air-Popped, No Butter)**: A low-fat, high-fiber snack option.
44. **Potatoes**: Low in acid and can be a soothing food option.
45. **Pumpkin**: Low in acid and high in fiber, which can help manage reflux.
46. **Quinoa**: A high-fiber grain that can help manage reflux.
47. **Radishes**: Low in acid and can help manage reflux symptoms.
48. **Rice Cakes**: Low in fat and can be a good snack option for those with acid reflux.
49. **Salmon**: High in omega-3 fatty acids, which have anti-inflammatory properties.
50. **Seafood**: Generally low in fat, making it a good protein option for those with acid reflux.
51. **Skim Milk**: Low in fat and can be soothing to the digestive tract.
52. **Sweet Potatoes**: Low in acid and high in fiber, they can help manage reflux symptoms.
53. **Tofu**: A low-fat protein option that can help manage reflux symptoms.
54. **Tuna (In Water)**: A low-fat protein option that can be easy on the stomach.
55. **Turkey Broth (Low-Fat)**: Similar to chicken broth, it is a low-fat and soothing option.
56. **Turnips**: Low in acid and can be a good addition to a reflux-friendly diet.
57. **White Fish (Cod, Haddock)**: Low in fat and a good source of lean protein.
58. **Whole Grains (Brown Rice, Quinoa)**: High in fiber, they help absorb stomach acid and reduce reflux symptoms.
59. **Zucchini**: Low in acid and can be easily digested.

60.

ACIDIC PH TABLE OF FOODS

pH is a measure of how acidic or alkaline a substance is, ranging from 0 to 14. A pH of 7 is considered neutral, below 7 is acidic, and above 7 is alkaline. The pH scale is logarithmic, meaning each whole number on the scale represents a tenfold difference in acidity or alkalinity. For instance, a substance with a pH of 4 is ten times more acidic than one with a pH of 5.

Foods with a lower pH (acidic foods) can exacerbate acid reflux symptoms by increasing the acidity in the stomach and esophagus. Conversely, foods with a higher pH (alkaline foods) can help neutralize stomach acid and reduce reflux symptoms.

Below is a table of common ingredients used in our recipes, categorized by their pH values. This table will help you make informed decisions about which foods to include in your diet to better manage acid reflux.

Acidic pH Table of Common Ingredients

Ingredient	pH Value
Apples	3.3 - 4.0
Avocado	6.3 - 6.6
Bananas	4.5 - 5.2
Blueberries	3.1 - 3.3
Broccoli	6.3 - 6.8
Carrots	5.8 - 6.3
Cauliflower	5.6 - 6.0
Celery	5.7 - 6.0
Chickpeas	6.0 - 6.6
Greek Yogurt	4.0 - 4.4
Green Beans	5.6 - 6.2
Kale	6.0 - 6.8
Lean Chicken (cooked)	5.8 - 6.0
Lentils	6.3 - 6.8
Oatmeal	6.2 - 6.6
Olive Oil	6.0 - 7.0
Potatoes	5.4 - 5.9
Quinoa	6.0 - 6.5
Spinach	5.5 - 6.8
Sweet Potatoes	5.3 - 5.6
Tuna (cooked)	5.9 - 6.1
Turkey (cooked)	5.8 - 6.2
Zucchini	5.6 - 6.1

Notes:
- **Apples**: The pH can vary depending on the variety and ripeness of the apple.
- **Avocado**: Generally more alkaline, making it a safe choice for those with acid reflux.
- **Bananas**: Slightly acidic but generally well-tolerated by those with acid reflux.
- **Blueberries**: Quite acidic; should be consumed in moderation by those with severe acid reflux.
- **Broccoli and Kale**: Both are relatively alkaline and safe for acid reflux.
- **Greek Yogurt**: Despite its acidity, it is often well-tolerated due to its probiotic content.

- **Oatmeal**: Neutral to slightly alkaline, making it a great choice for acid reflux sufferers.
- **Olive Oil**: Neutral to alkaline, a safe fat option for acid reflux.

Understanding the pH levels of these common ingredients can guide you in making dietary choices that help manage and alleviate the symptoms of acid reflux. By selecting more alkaline foods and avoiding highly acidic ones, you can create a diet that supports better digestive health and reduces discomfort.

Chapter 03

ACID REFLUX DIET COOKBOOK

t's time to deliver on our promise. In this cookbook, you will find a diverse selection of over 70 recipes, spanning from hearty breakfasts to delectable desserts. Start your day with recipes like Banana Oat Pancakes and Quinoa Breakfast Bowls that provide the energy and nutrients you need without triggering acid reflux. For lunch, enjoy satisfying options such as Grilled Chicken and Vegetable Wraps or Lentil and Spinach Salads that keep your midday meal light and refreshing.

Dinner recipes like Herb-Roasted Chicken with Carrots and Potatoes and Mushroom and Barley Soup offer comforting and filling choices that won't compromise your evening. Our collection of soups includes soothing options like Sweet Potato and Black Bean Soup, perfect for a cozy meal any time of the year. Additionally, our salad recipes, such as the Cucumber and Dill Salad, provide crisp and flavorful choices for those seeking a lighter fare.

Snacks and hors d'oeuvres are covered with tasty, reflux-friendly options like Zucchini Chips and Chickpea and Avocado Mash on Whole Grain Toast, ensuring you have healthy bites between meals. Finally, our dessert section allows you to indulge your sweet tooth with treats like Chia Seed Pudding and Strawberry Almond Parfait, offering a satisfying end to your meal without the worry of acid reflux symptoms. Each recipe is crafted to minimize acidity and promote digestive health, helping you enjoy your meals and improve your quality of life.

BREAKFAST RECIPES

Start your day with a reflux-free nutritious breakfast. Our selection of breakfast recipes focuses on incorporating ingredients that are gentle and provide the essential nutrients to kickstart your day. Each recipe is designed to minimize acid production and avoid common reflux triggers, ensuring a smooth and enjoyable morning meal that supports your overall health.

OATMEAL WITH BANANAS AND ALMONDS

Difficulty:	**Prep Time:**	**Cooking Method:**	**Servings:**
Easy	5 minutes	Stovetop	2

INGREDIENTS:

- 1 cup steel-cut oatmeal
- 2 cups water or skim milk
- 1 banana, sliced
- A handful of almonds, chopped

INSTRUCTIONS:

1. **Start by bringing the water or skim milk** to a gentle boil in a pot. Add the oatmeal and reduce the heat, letting it simmer. Stir occasionally to prevent sticking and ensure even cooking.

2. **Once the oatmeal reaches a creamy consistency,** serve it into bowls. Arrange the sliced bananas on top and sprinkle with chopped almonds for added texture and nutrients.

NUTRITIONAL VALUES (PER SERVING):

- Calories: 210
- Protein: 6g
- Carbohydrates: 38g
- Fat: 5g
- Fiber: 5g
- Sugar: 10g

GREEK YOGURT WITH HONEY AND PEARS

Difficulty:
Easy

Prep Time:
5 minutes

Cooking Method:
None

Servings:
2

INGREDIENTS:

- 1 cup low-fat Greek yogurt
- 1 pear, sliced
- 1 tablespoon honey

INSTRUCTIONS:

1. Spoon the Greek yogurt into two bowls.
2. **Arrange the pear slices** on top of the yogurt, distributing them evenly.
3. **Drizzle each serving with honey.** Enjoy this refreshing and nutritious breakfast, perfect for managing acid reflux while providing essential nutrients and probiotics.

NUTRITIONAL VALUES (PER SERVING):

- Calories: 180
- Protein: 12g
- Carbohydrates: 26g
- Fat: 2g
- Fiber: 3g
- Sugar: 20g

SCRAMBLED EGG WHITES WITH SPINACH

| Difficulty:
Easy | Prep Time:
5 minutes | Cooking Method:
Stovetop | Servings:
2 |

INGREDIENTS:

- 4 egg whites
- 1 cup fresh spinach, chopped
- 1 tablespoon olive oil
- Salt and pepper to taste

INSTRUCTIONS:

1. **Heat the olive oil** in a non-stick skillet over medium heat. Add the chopped spinach and sauté until wilted.
2. **Pour in the egg whites**, stirring gently. Cook until the egg whites are set and fully cooked, seasoning with salt and pepper to taste.
3. cooked, seasoning with salt and pepper to taste.
4. **Serve hot**, enjoying a protein-packed, low-fat breakfast that's easy on the stomach and ideal for managing acid reflux.

NUTRITIONAL VALUES(PER SERVING):

- Calories: 80
- Protein: 12g
- Carbohydrates: 1g
- Fat: 3g
- Fiber: 1g
- Sugar: 0g

AVOCADO AND TURKEY BREAKFAST WRAP

Difficulty:	**Prep Time:**	**Cooking Method:**	**Servings:**
Easy	10 minutes	None	2

INGREDIENTS:

- 2 whole grain wraps
- 1 avocado, mashed
- 4 slices turkey breast
- 1/2 cup shredded lettuce
- 1/2 cucumber, thinly sliced

INSTRUCTIONS:

1. **Spread the mashed avocado** evenly over each whole grain wrap.
2. **Layer the turkey slices**, shredded lettuce, and cucumber slices on top.
3. **Roll up the wraps**, cut in half, and enjoy a nutritious and filling breakfast that's gentle on the stomach and supports digestive health.

NUTRITIONAL VALUES (PER SERVING):

- Calories: 300
- Protein: 15g
- Carbohydrates: 28g
- Fat: 15g
- Fiber: 7g
- Sugar: 2g

BANANA AND OAT SMOOTHIE

Difficulty:	Prep Time:	Cooking Method:	Servings:
Easy	**5 minutes**	**Blender**	**2**

INGREDIENTS:

- 1 banana
- 1/2 cup rolled oats
- 1 cup hemp milk
- 1 teaspoon honey
- 1/2 teaspoon cinnamon

INSTRUCTIONS:

1. **Combine the banana**, rolled oats, hemp milk, honey, and cinnamon in a blender.

2. **Blend until smooth and creamy.** Pour into glasses and enjoy a quick, nutritious breakfast that's perfect for managing acid reflux.

NUTRITIONAL VALUES (PER SERVING):

- Calories: 200
- Protein: 4g
- Carbohydrates: 38g
- Fat: 4g
- Fiber: 4g
- Sugar: 12g

QUINOA BREAKFAST BOWL WITH BERRIES

Difficulty:	Prep Time:	Cooking Method:	Servings:
Easy	10 minutes	Stovetop	2

INGREDIENTS:

- 1 cup cooked quinoa
- 1/2 cup fresh berries (blueberries, strawberries, or raspberries)
- 1/2 cup hemp milk
- 1 tablespoon chia seeds
- 1 teaspoon honey

INSTRUCTIONS:

1. **Cook the quinoa** according to package instructions and let it cool slightly.
2. **Divide the cooked quinoa** into two bowls. Top with fresh berries and chia seeds.
3. **Pour hemp milk** over the mixture and drizzle with honey. Enjoy a refreshing and nutrient-packed breakfast that supports digestive health and helps manage acid reflux.

NUTRITIONAL VALUES (PER SERVING):

- Calories: 220
- Protein: 6g
- Carbohydrates: 38g
- Fat: 6g
- Fiber: 6g
- Sugar: 10g

APPLE CHIA PUDDING

Difficulty:	Prep Time:	Cooking Method:	Servings:
Easy	5 minutes (plus overnight refrigeration)	None	2

INGREDIENTS:

- 1/4 cup chia seeds
- 1 cup hemp milk
- 1 apple, diced
- 1/2 teaspoon cinnamon
- 1 teaspoon honey

INSTRUCTIONS:

1. **In a bowl,** mix chia seeds and hemp milk. Stir well to avoid clumping.
2. **Add diced apple and cinnamon,** then mix in honey.
3. **Cover and refrigerate overnight.** In the morning, give it a good stir and enjoy a delicious, fiber-rich breakfast that's gentle on your stomach.

NUTRITIONAL VALUES (PER SERVING):

- Calories: 180
- Protein: 4g
- Carbohydrates: 30g
- Fat: 7g
- Fiber: 10g
- Sugar: 14g

WHOLE GRAIN TOAST WITH ALMOND BUTTER AND SLICED BANANAS

Difficulty: Easy	Prep Time: 5 minutes	Cooking Method: Toaster	Servings: 2

INGREDIENTS:

- 2 slices whole grain bread
- 2 tablespoons almond butter
- 1 banana, sliced

INSTRUCTIONS:

1. **Toast the whole grain bread** to your desired level of crispness.
2. **Spread a tablespoon** of almond butter on each slice of toast.
3. **Top with banana slices.** This quick and nutritious breakfast is perfect for managing acid reflux while providing essential nutrients.

NUTRITIONAL VALUES (PER SERVING):

- Calories: 250
- Protein: 7g
- Carbohydrates: 36g
- Fat: 10g
- Fiber: 6g
- Sugar: 10g

STRAWBERRY AND SPINACH SMOOTHIE

Difficulty:	Prep Time:	Cooking Method:	Servings:
Easy	5 minutes	Blender	2

INGREDIENTS:

- 1 cup fresh spinach
- 1 cup fresh strawberries
- 1 banana
- 1 cup hemp milk
- 1 teaspoon honey

INSTRUCTIONS:

1. **Combine spinach**, strawberries, banana, almond milk, and honey in a blender.

2. **Blend until smooth and creamy.** Pour into glasses and enjoy a nutrient-dense breakfast that's easy on the digestive system and helps manage acid reflux.

NUTRITIONAL VALUES (PER SERVING):

- Calories: 180
- Protein: 3g
- Carbohydrates: 39g
- Fat: 3g
- Fiber: 5g
- Sugar: 25g

COTTAGE CHEESE WITH MELON AND ALMONDS

Difficulty:
Easy

Prep Time:
5 minutes

Cooking Method:
None

Servings:
2

INGREDIENTS:

- 1 cup low-fat cottage cheese
- 1 cup diced melon (cantaloupe or honeydew)
- A handful of almonds, chopped

INSTRUCTIONS:

1. **Spoon the cottage cheese** into two bowls.
2. **Top with diced melon** and a sprinkle of chopped almonds. This simple and refreshing breakfast provides protein and essential nutrients while being gentle on the stomach.

NUTRITIONAL VALUES (PER SERVING):

- Calories: 200
- Protein: 14g
- Carbohydrates: 18g
- Fat: 7g
- Fiber: 2g
- Sugar: 12g

LUNCH RECIPES

Midday meals help maintain energy levels and keep acid reflux at bay. Our lunch recipes are crafted to offer balanced, reflux-friendly options that combine lean proteins, whole grains, and a variety of vegetables. These recipes will nourish your body as well as help in controlling acid production, making your afternoon both productive and comfortable.

GRILLED CHICKEN AND QUINOA SALAD

Difficulty:	Prep Time:	Cooking Method:	Servings:
Easy	15 minutes	Grilling and Stovetop	2

INGREDIENTS:

- 1 cup quinoa
- 2 cups water or low-sodium chicken broth
- 1 grilled chicken breast, sliced
- 2 cups mixed greens
- 1/2 cucumber, sliced
- 2 tablespoons olive oil
- Salt and pepper to taste

INSTRUCTIONS:

1. **Cook the quinoa** by bringing water or chicken broth to a boil in a pot. Add the quinoa, reduce heat, cover, and simmer for about 15 minutes or until the liquid is absorbed. Fluff with a fork and let cool.
2. **Grill the chicken breast** until fully cooked, then slice into thin strips.
3. **Assemble the salad** by combining the mixed greens, cucumber, and quinoa in a large bowl.
4. **Top with grilled chicken slices.**
5. **Drizzle with olive oil,** then season with salt and pepper to taste.
6. **Enjoy this refreshing salad** that is gentle on your stomach and helps manage acid reflux.

NUTRITIONAL VALUES (PER SERVING):

- Calories: 350
- Protein: 28g
- Carbohydrates: 30g
- Fat: 12g
- Fiber: 5g
- Sugar: 4g

CHICKPEA AND AVOCADO WRAPS

Difficulty:	Prep Time:	Cooking Method:	Servings:
Easy	**10 minutes**	**None**	**2**

INGREDIENTS:

- 1 can chickpeas, drained and rinsed
- 1 ripe avocado, mashed
- 1 cup fresh spinach
- 1/2 cup shredded carrots
- 1/2 teaspoon cumin
- Juice of 1 lime
- Salt and pepper to taste
- 2 whole grain tortillas

INSTRUCTIONS:

1. **In a bowl**, combine the chickpeas, mashed avocado, cumin, lime juice, salt, and pepper. Mix until well combined.
2. **Lay out the tortillas** and evenly distribute the spinach and shredded carrots.
3. **Spoon the chickpea** and avocado mixture onto the tortillas.
4. **Roll up the tortillas tightly**, securing with a toothpick if necessary.
5. **Serve immediately** or wrap in foil for a convenient on-the-go meal.

NUTRITIONAL VALUES (PER SERVING):

- Calories: 320
- Protein: 10g
- Carbohydrates: 45g
- Fat: 12g
- Fiber: 12g
- Sugar: 4g

BAKED SALMON WITH ASPARAGUS

Difficulty:	Prep Time:	Cooking Method:	Servings:
Easy	**10 minutes**	**Oven**	**2**

INGREDIENTS:

- 2 salmon fillets
- 1 bunch asparagus, trimmed
- 2 tablespoons olive oil
- Salt and pepper to taste

INSTRUCTIONS:

1. **Preheat the oven** to 400°F (200°C).
2. **Place the salmon fillets** on a baking sheet lined with parchment paper.
3. **Arrange the asparagus** around the salmon.
4. **Drizzle olive oil** over the salmon and asparagus.
5. **Season with salt and pepper.**
6. **Bake for 15-20 minutes**, or until the salmon is cooked through and the asparagus is tender.
7. **Enjoy** this healthy and delicious meal that's perfect for managing acid reflux.

NUTRITIONAL VALUES (PER SERVING):

- Calories: 350
- Protein: 35g
- Carbohydrates: 6g
- Fat: 20g
- Fiber: 3g
- Sugar: 2g

VEGETABLE AND TOFU STIR-FRY

Difficulty:	Prep Time:	Cooking Method:	Servings:
Easy	15 minutes	Stovetop	2

INGREDIENTS:

- 1 block firm tofu, drained and cubed
- 1 cup broccoli florets
- 1 cup green beans, trimmed
- 1 zucchini, sliced
- 2 tablespoons olive oil
- 2 tablespoons low-sodium soy sauce
- 1 teaspoon grated ginger
- 1 tablespoon honey (optional)
- Salt and pepper to taste

INSTRUCTIONS:

1. **Heat the olive oil** in a large skillet over medium heat. Add the cubed tofu and cook until golden brown, then remove from the skillet and set aside.

2. Add the **broccoli, green beans, and zucchini** to the skillet and stir-fry for about 5-7 minutes, until the vegetables are tender-crisp.
   Return the tofu to the skillet and stir in the soy sauce, grated ginger, and honey if using.

3. **Season with salt and pepper** to taste and cook for another 2-3 minutes.

4. **Serve immediately** and enjoy a nutritious, acid reflux-friendly meal.

NUTRITIONAL VALUES (PER SERVING):

- Calories: 280
- Protein: 16g
- Carbohydrates: 20g
- Fat: 18g
- Fiber: 5g
- Sugar: 8g

CHICKEN AND SWEET POTATO SALAD

Difficulty:	Prep Time:	Cooking Method:	Servings:
Easy	10 minutes	Stovetop and Oven	2

INGREDIENTS:

- 1 grilled chicken breast, sliced
- 2 medium sweet potatoes, peeled and cubed
- 2 cups fresh spinach
- 2 tablespoons olive oil
- Salt and pepper to taste

INSTRUCTIONS:

1. **Preheat the oven** to 400°F (200°C).
2. **Toss the sweet potato cubes** with 1 tablespoon of olive oil, salt, and pepper. Spread them on a baking sheet and roast for 20-25 minutes, until tender.
3. **In a large bowl, combine the fresh spinach**, grilled chicken slices, and roasted sweet potatoes.
4. **Drizzle with the remaining olive oil** and toss gently to combine.
5. **Season with salt and pepper to taste.** Enjoy this hearty and nutritious salad that helps manage acid reflux.

NUTRITIONAL VALUES (PER SERVING):

- Calories: 350
- Protein: 28g
- Carbohydrates: 35g
- Fat: 12g
- Fiber: 6g
- Sugar: 10g

TURKEY AND SPINACH SALAD

Difficulty:	Prep Time:	Cooking Method:	Servings:
Easy	**10 minutes**	**None**	**2**

INGREDIENTS:

- 4 cups fresh spinach leaves
- 4 slices turkey breast, chopped
- 1/2 cucumber, sliced
- 1/4 cup chopped almonds
- 2 tablespoons olive oil
- Salt and pepper to taste

INSTRUCTIONS:

1. **Combine the fresh spinach leaves**, chopped turkey, cucumber slices, and chopped almonds in a large bowl.

2. **Drizzle with olive oil** and toss gently to combine.
3. **Season with salt and pepper to taste.**
4. **Enjoy** this light and refreshing salad that supports digestive health and helps manage acid reflux.

NUTRITIONAL VALUES (PER SERVING):

- Calories: 250
- Protein: 20g
- Carbohydrates: 8g
- Fat: 16g
- Fiber: 3g
- Sugar: 2g

GRILLED SHRIMP AND ZUCCHINI SKEWERS

Difficulty:	Prep Time:	Cooking Method:	Servings:
Easy	**10 minutes**	**Grilling**	**2**

INGREDIENTS:

- 12 large shrimp, peeled and deveined
- 2 zucchinis, sliced into rounds
- 2 tablespoons olive oil
- 1 teaspoon grated ginger
- Salt and pepper to taste

INSTRUCTIONS:

1. **Preheat the grill** to medium-high heat.
2. **Thread the shrimp and zucchini** slices onto skewers.
3. **Brush with olive oil** and sprinkle with grated ginger, salt, and pepper.
4. **Grill for 2-3 minutes per side**, or until the shrimp are opaque and the zucchini is tender.
5. **Serve hot and enjoy** a nutritious meal that's gentle on your stomach.

NUTRITIONAL VALUES (PER SERVING):

- Calories: 200
- Protein: 22g
- Carbohydrates: 6g
- Fat: 10g
- Fiber: 2g
- Sugar: 2g

LENTIL AND VEGETABLE STEW

Difficulty:	Prep Time:	Cooking Method:	Servings:
Easy	**15 minutes**	**Stovetop**	**2**

INGREDIENTS:

- 1 cup lentils, rinsed
- 1 carrot, diced
- 1 celery stalk, diced
- 1 fennel bulb, diced
- 4 cups low-sodium vegetable broth
- 2 tablespoons olive oil
- 1 teaspoon dried thyme
- Salt and pepper to taste

INSTRUCTIONS:

1. **Heat olive oil** in a large pot over medium heat. Add the carrot, celery, and fennel, and cook until softened.

2. **Add the lentils, vegetable broth, and dried thyme.** Bring to a boil, then reduce heat and simmer for 25-30 minutes, or until the lentils are tender.

3. **Season with salt and pepper to taste. Serve hot** and enjoy this hearty, nutrient-dense stew that supports digestive health.

NUTRITIONAL VALUES (PER SERVING):

- Calories: 300
- Protein: 16g
- Carbohydrates: 45g
- Fat: 10g
- Fiber: 16g
- Sugar: 8g

GRILLED CHICKEN WITH STEAMED BROCCOLI

Difficulty:	Prep Time:	Cooking Method:	Servings:
Easy	10 minutes	Grilling and Steaming	2

INGREDIENTS:

- 2 grilled chicken breasts
- 2 cups broccoli florets
- 1 tablespoon olive oil
- Salt and pepper to taste

INSTRUCTIONS:

1. **Preheat the grill to medium-high heat.**
2. **Grill the chicken breasts** until fully cooked, about 6-8 minutes per side.
3. **Steam the broccoli** florets until tender, about 5 minutes.
4. **Drizzle olive oil** over the steamed broccoli and season with salt and pepper.
5. **Serve the grilled chicken** with the steamed broccoli and enjoy a simple, nutritious meal that helps manage acid reflux.

NUTRITIONAL VALUES (PER SERVING):

- Calories: 300
- Protein: 35g
- Carbohydrates: 10g
- Fat: 12g
- Fiber: 4g
- Sugar: 2g

TUNA SALAD WITH CUCUMBER AND GREEK YOGURT

Difficulty:	Prep Time:	Cooking Method:	Servings:
Easy	10 minutes	None	2

INGREDIENTS:

- 1 can tuna in water, drained
- 1/2 cucumber, diced
- 1/2 cup low-fat Greek yogurt
- 1 tablespoon chopped fresh parsley
- Salt and pepper to taste

INSTRUCTIONS:

1. **In a bowl**, combine the drained tuna, diced cucumber, and Greek yogurt.
2. **Stir in the chopped parsley** and season with salt and pepper.
3. **Serve immediately and enjoy** a light, protein-rich lunch that's gentle on your stomach and supports digestive health.

NUTRITIONAL VALUES (PER SERVING):

- Calories: 200
- Protein: 28g
- Carbohydrates: 6g
- Fat: 6g
- Fiber: 1g
- Sugar: 4g

DINNER
RECIPES

BAKED COD WITH GREEN BEANS

Difficulty:	Prep Time:	Cooking Method:	Servings:
Easy	10 minutes	Oven	2

INGREDIENTS:

- 2 cod fillets
- 2 cups green beans, trimmed
- 2 tablespoons olive oil
- 1 teaspoon dried thyme
- Salt and pepper to taste

INSTRUCTIONS:

1. Preheat the oven to 400°F (200°C).
2. **Place the cod fillets** on a baking sheet lined with parchment paper. Arrange the green beans around the fish.
3. **Drizzle olive oil** over the cod and green beans. Sprinkle with dried thyme, salt, and pepper.
4. **Bake for 15-20 minutes**, or until the cod is cooked through and the green beans are tender.
5. **Serve hot and enjoy** a nutritious, acid reflux-friendly dinner.

NUTRITIONAL VALUES (PER SERVING):

- Calories: 280
- Protein: 30g
- Carbohydrates: 8g
- Fat: 14g
- Fiber: 4g
- Sugar: 4g

GRILLED CHICKEN AND SWEET POTATO MASH

Difficulty:	Prep Time:	Cooking Method:	Servings:
Easy	15 minutes	Grilling and Stovetop	2

INGREDIENTS:

- 2 chicken breasts
- 2 medium sweet potatoes, peeled and cubed
- 2 tablespoons olive oil
- 1 teaspoon dried rosemary
- Salt and pepper to taste

INSTRUCTIONS:

1. **Preheat the grill** to medium-high heat.
2. **Grill the chicken** breasts for about 6-8 minutes per side, or until fully cooked.
3. **Boil the sweet potatoes** in a pot of water until tender, about 10-15 minutes. Drain and mash with olive oil, rosemary, salt, and pepper.
4. **Serve the grilled chicken** alongside the sweet potato mash for a balanced and soothing dinner.

NUTRITIONAL VALUES (PER SERVING):

- Calories: 400
- Protein: 35g
- Carbohydrates: 35g
- Fat: 14g
- Fiber: 6g
- Sugar: 8g

SEARED SCALLOPS WITH SPINACH AND QUINOA

Difficulty:	Prep Time:	Cooking Method:	Servings:
Moderate	**20 minutes**	**Stovetop**	**2**

INGREDIENTS:

- 10 large scallops
- 1 cup quinoa
- 2 cups water or low-sodium vegetable broth
- 4 cups fresh spinach
- 2 tablespoons olive oil
- Salt and pepper to taste

INSTRUCTIONS:

1. **Cook the quinoa** by bringing water or broth to a boil. Add quinoa, reduce heat, cover, and simmer for about 15 minutes until liquid is absorbed.
2. **Heat 1 tablespoon of olive oil** in a skillet over medium-high heat. Sear the scallops for 2-3 minutes on each side until golden. Remove and set aside.
3. **In the same skillet, add the remaining olive oil** and sauté the spinach until wilted. Season with salt and pepper.
4. **Serve the scallops over a bed of quinoa** with spinach on the side for a nutrient-rich dinner.

NUTRITIONAL VALUES (PER SERVING):

- Calories: 350
- Protein: 25g
- Carbohydrates: 35g
- Fat: 14g
- Fiber: 6g
- Sugar: 3g

CHICKEN AND VEGETABLE STIR-FRY

Difficulty:	**Prep Time:**	**Cooking Method:**	**Servings:**
Easy	15 minutes	Stovetop	2

INGREDIENTS:

- 2 chicken breasts, sliced
- 1 cup broccoli florets
- 1 zucchini, sliced
- 1 carrot, sliced
- 2 tablespoons olive oil
- 2 tablespoons low-sodium soy sauce
- 1 teaspoon grated ginger
- Salt and pepper to taste

INSTRUCTIONS:

1. **Heat olive oil** in a large skillet over medium-high heat. Add the sliced chicken and cook until browned, then remove and set aside.

2. **Add the broccoli, zucchini, and carrot** to the skillet and stir-fry until tender-crisp.

3. **Return the chicken to the skillet** and add the soy sauce and grated ginger. Stir well and cook for another 2-3 minutes.

4. **Season with salt and pepper** to taste and serve immediately for a quick, healthy dinner.

NUTRITIONAL VALUES (PER SERVING):

- Calories: 300
- Protein: 30g
- Carbohydrates: 15g
- Fat: 14g
- Fiber: 5g
- Sugar: 6g

BROILED TILAPIA WITH STEAMED BROCCOLI

Difficulty:	Prep Time:	Cooking Method:	Servings:
Easy	10 minutes	Broiling and Steaming	2

INGREDIENTS:

- 2 tilapia fillets
- 2 cups broccoli florets
- 2 tablespoons olive oil
- 1 teaspoon dried basil
- Salt and pepper to taste

INSTRUCTIONS:

1. **Preheat the broiler.**
2. **Place the tilapia fillets** on a baking sheet lined with aluminum foil. Drizzle with olive oil and sprinkle with dried basil, salt, and pepper.
3. **Broil the tilapia for 5-7 minutes,** or until the fish is cooked through and flakes easily with a fork.
4. **Steam the broccoli** until tender, about 5 minutes.
5. **Serve the broiled tilapia** with steamed broccoli for a light, healthy dinner that supports digestive health.

NUTRITIONAL VALUES (PER SERVING):

- Calories: 250
- Protein: 30g
- Carbohydrates: 8g
- Fat: 12g
- Fiber: 4g
- Sugar: 2g

HERB-ROASTED CHICKEN WITH CARROTS AND POTATOES

Difficulty:
Easy

Prep Time:
15 minutes

Cooking Method:
Oven

Servings:
2

INGREDIENTS:

- 2 chicken breasts
- 2 medium potatoes, cubed
- 2 large carrots, sliced
- 2 tablespoons olive oil
- 1 teaspoon dried rosemary
- 1 teaspoon dried thyme
- Salt and pepper to taste

INSTRUCTIONS:

1. Preheat the oven to 400°F (200°C).
2. **Toss the potatoes** and carrots with 1 tablespoon of olive oil, rosemary, thyme, salt, and pepper. Spread them on a baking sheet.
3. **Place the chicken breasts** on top of the vegetables and drizzle with the remaining olive oil. Season with additional salt and pepper.
4. **Roast for 25-30 minutes**, or until the chicken is cooked through and the vegetables are tender.
5. **Serve hot and enjoy** a wholesome, balanced meal.

NUTRITIONAL VALUES (PER SERVING):

- Calories: 450
- Protein: 35g
- Carbohydrates: 35g
- Fat: 18g
- Fiber: 6g
- Sugar: 7g

QUINOA AND BLACK BEAN BOWLS

Difficulty:	Prep Time:	Cooking Method:	Servings:
Easy	**15 minutes**	**Stovetop**	**2**

INGREDIENTS:

- 1 cup quinoa
- 2 cups low-sodium vegetable broth
- 1 can black beans, drained and rinsed
- 1 cup corn kernels (fresh or frozen)
- 1 ripe avocado, diced
- 1 zucchini, diced
- Juice of 1 lime (if tolerated, or omit)
- 1 tablespoon olive oil
- 1 teaspoon ground cumin
- Salt and pepper to taste
- Fresh cilantro, chopped (for garnish)

INSTRUCTIONS:

1. Rinse the quinoa under cold water. In a medium saucepan, combine the quinoa and vegetable broth. Bring to a boil, then reduce the heat to low, cover, and simmer for about 15 minutes or until the quinoa is cooked and the liquid is absorbed.

2. **In a large bowl**, combine the cooked quinoa, black beans, corn, avocado, and zucchini.
3. **In a small bowl**, whisk together the olive oil, ground cumin, salt, and pepper.
4. **Pour the dressing** over the quinoa mixture and toss to combine.
5. **Garnish with fresh cilantro.**
6. **Serve immediately,** or refrigerate for a cold salad.

NUTRITIONAL VALUES (PER SERVING):

- Calories: 350
- Protein: 12g
- Carbohydrates: 50g
- Fat: 13g
- Fiber: 12g
- Sugar: 5g

GRILLED TURKEY BURGERS WITH AVOCADO

Difficulty:
Easy

Prep Time:
10 minutes

Cooking Method:
Grilling

Servings:
2

INGREDIENTS:

- 2 turkey burger patties
- 2 whole grain burger buns
- 1 avocado, sliced
- 2 leaves lettuce
- 2 tablespoons olive oil
- Salt and pepper to taste

INSTRUCTIONS:

1. Preheat the grill to medium-high heat.
2. **Brush the turkey patties** with olive oil and season with salt and pepper.
3. **Grill the patties** for about 5-6 minutes per side, or until fully cooked.
4. **Toast the burger buns** on the grill for a minute or until slightly crispy.
5. **Assemble the burgers** by placing a turkey patty on each bun, topping with lettuce and avocado slices.
6. **Serve hot and enjoy** a nutritious, acid reflux-friendly dinner.

NUTRITIONAL VALUES (PER SERVING):

- Calories: 400
- Protein: 30g
- Carbohydrates: 28g
- Fat: 20g
- Fiber: 8g
- Sugar: 2g

CHICKPEA AND SPINACH STEW

Difficulty:
Easy

Prep Time:
15 minutes

Cooking Method:
Stovetop

Servings:
2

INGREDIENTS:

- 1 can chickpeas, drained and rinsed
- 4 cups fresh spinach
- 1 cup chopped celery
- 2 tablespoons olive oil
- 4 cups low-sodium vegetable broth
- 1 teaspoon ground cumin
- Salt and pepper to taste

INSTRUCTIONS:

1. **Heat olive oil** in a large pot over medium heat. Add the chopped celery and cook until softened.
2. **Stir in the chickpeas** and ground cumin. Cook for a couple of minutes until fragrant.
3. **Add the vegetable broth** and bring to a simmer. Cook for 10 minutes.
4. **Stir in the fresh spinach** and cook until wilted. Season with salt and pepper.
5. **Serve hot** and enjoy a hearty and nutritious stew.

NUTRITIONAL VALUES (PER SERVING):

- Calories: 300
- Protein: 12g
- Carbohydrates: 40g
- Fat: 12g
- Fiber: 10g
- Sugar: 6g

MUSHROOM AND QUINOA PILAF

Difficulty:	Prep Time:	Cooking Method:	Servings:
Easy	15 minutes	Stovetop	2

INGREDIENTS:

- 1 cup quinoa
- 2 cups low-sodium vegetable broth
- 1 cup mushrooms, sliced
- 1 cup chopped celery
- 2 tablespoons olive oil
- 1 teaspoon dried thyme
- Salt and pepper to taste

INSTRUCTIONS:

1. **Cook the quinoa** by bringing vegetable broth to a boil. Add quinoa, reduce heat, cover, and simmer for about 15 minutes until liquid is absorbed.

2. **Heat olive oil** in a skillet over medium heat. Add the chopped celery and sliced mushrooms. Cook until the vegetables are tender.

3. **Stir in the cooked quinoa** and dried thyme. Season with salt and pepper.

4. **Serve hot** and enjoy a flavorful and nutritious pilaf.

NUTRITIONAL VALUES (PER SERVING):

- Calories: 320
- Protein: 10g
- Carbohydrates: 45g
- Fat: 12g
- Fiber: 8g
- Sugar: 4g

SALAD
RECIPES

Salads are a refreshing way to manage acid reflux. Our salad recipes focus on combining nutrient-dense ingredients that are low in acidity and gentle on the stomach, offering a delightful mix of flavors and textures while providing a light yet satisfying option for meals or side dishes that support your digestive health.

AVOCADO AND CHICKEN SALAD

Difficulty:	Prep Time:	Cooking Method:	Servings:
Easy	10 minutes	None	2

INGREDIENTS:

- 1 grilled chicken breast, diced
- 1 avocado, diced
- 2 cups mixed greens
- 1/2 cucumber, sliced
- 1/2 cup shredded carrots
- 2 tablespoons olive oil
- Salt and pepper to taste

INSTRUCTIONS:

1. **In a large bowl, combine** the diced chicken, avocado, mixed greens, cucumber, and shredded carrots.
2. **Drizzle with olive oil** and season with salt and pepper.
3. **Toss gently** to combine.
4. **Serve immediately** and enjoy a refreshing, nutritious salad.

NUTRITIONAL VALUES (PER SERVING):

- Calories: 320
- Protein: 20g
- Carbohydrates: 18g
- Fat: 20g
- Fiber: 10g
- Sugar: 4g

KALE AND APPLE SALAD

Difficulty:	**Prep Time:**	**Cooking Method:**	**Servings:**
Easy	**10 minutes**	**None**	**2**

INGREDIENTS:

- 2 cups chopped kale
- 1 apple, thinly sliced
- 1/4 cup walnuts, chopped
- 1/4 cup dried cranberries
- 2 tablespoons olive oil
- 1 tablespoon honey
- Salt to taste

INSTRUCTIONS:

1. **In a large bowl, combine** the kale, apple slices, walnuts, and dried cranberries.
2. **Drizzle with olive oil and honey,** then season with salt.
3. **Toss well** to combine.
4. **Serve immediately** and enjoy a crunchy, sweet, and nutritious salad.

NUTRITIONAL VALUES (PER SERVING):

- Calories: 300
- Protein: 5g
- Carbohydrates: 35g
- Fat: 18g
- Fiber: 8g
- Sugar: 20g

TURKEY AND CRANBERRY SALAD

Difficulty:	Prep Time:	Cooking Method:	Servings:
Easy	10 minutes	None	2

INGREDIENTS:

- 1 cup sliced turkey breast
- 2 cups mixed greens
- 1/4 cup dried cranberries
- 1/4 cup chopped celery
- 2 tablespoons olive oil
- Salt and pepper to taste

INSTRUCTIONS:

1. **In a large bowl, combine** the turkey, mixed greens, dried cranberries, and chopped celery.
2. **Drizzle with olive oil** and season with salt and pepper.
3. **Toss gently** to combine.
4. **Serve immediately** and enjoy a flavorful, nutritious salad.

NUTRITIONAL VALUES (PER SERVING):

- Calories: 250
- Protein: 20g
- Carbohydrates: 15g
- Fat: 14g
- Fiber: 3g
- Sugar: 10g

LENTIL AND FETA SALAD

Difficulty:	Prep Time:	Cooking Method:	Servings:
Easy	**15 minutes**	**None**	**2**

INGREDIENTS:

- 1 cup cooked lentils
- 1/4 cup crumbled feta cheese (an allowed variety of cheese)
- 1/2 cucumber, diced
- 2 tablespoons chopped fresh parsley
- 2 tablespoons olive oil
- Salt and pepper to taste

INSTRUCTIONS:

1. **In a large bowl, combine** the lentils, feta cheese, cucumber, and parsley.
2. **Drizzle with olive oil** and season with salt and pepper.
3. **Toss gently** to combine.
4. **Serve immediately** and enjoy a protein-packed, nutritious salad.

NUTRITIONAL VALUES (PER SERVING):

- Calories: 300
- Protein: 15g
- Carbohydrates: 25g
- Fat: 16g
- Fiber: 10g
- Sugar: 4g

CUCUMBER AND DILL SALAD

Difficulty:	Prep Time:	Cooking Method:	Servings:
Easy	10 minutes	None	2

INGREDIENTS:

- 2 cups sliced cucumber
- 2 tablespoons fresh dill, chopped
- 1/4 cup low-fat Greek yogurt
- Salt to taste

INSTRUCTIONS:

1. **In a large bowl, combine** the sliced cucumber and chopped dill.
2. **Add the Greek yogurt** and mix well.
3. **Season with salt** to taste.
4. **Serve immediately** and enjoy a cool, refreshing salad.

NUTRITIONAL VALUES (PER SERVING):

- Calories: 100
- Protein: 5g
- Carbohydrates: 10g
- Fat: 4g
- Fiber: 2g
- Sugar: 6g

BROCCOLI AND CRANBERRY SALAD

9Difficulty:	Prep Time:	Cooking Method:	Servings:
Easy	10 minutes	None	2

INGREDIENTS:

- 2 cups steamed broccoli, cooled
- 1/4 cup dried cranberries
- 2 tablespoons sunflower seeds
- 2 tablespoons olive oil
- Salt and pepper to taste

INSTRUCTIONS:

1. **In a large bowl, combine** the steamed broccoli, dried cranberries, and sunflower seeds.
2. **Drizzle with olive oil** and season with salt and pepper.
3. **Toss gently** to combine.
4. **Serve immediately** and enjoy a nutritious, crunchy salad.

NUTRITIONAL VALUES (PER SERVING):

- Calories: 180
- Protein: 5g
- Carbohydrates: 20g
- Fat: 10g
- Fiber: 5g
- Sugar: 12g

CARROT AND RAISIN SALAD

Difficulty:	Prep Time:	Cooking Method:	Servings:
Easy	**10 minutes**	**None**	**2**

INGREDIENTS:

- 2 cups shredded carrots
- 1/4 cup raisins
- 2 tablespoons chopped parsley
- 1/4 cup low-fat Greek yogurt
- 1 tablespoon honey

INSTRUCTIONS:

1. **In a large bowl, combine** the shredded carrots, raisins, and chopped parsley.

2. **Add the Greek yogurt** and honey, then mix well.
3. **Serve immediately** and enjoy a sweet and tangy salad.

NUTRITIONAL VALUES (PER SERVING):

- Calories: 150
- Protein: 3g
- Carbohydrates: 30g
- Fat: 2g
- Fiber: 4g
- Sugar: 20g

FENNEL AND APPLE SALAD

Difficulty:	Prep Time:	Cooking Method:	Servings:
Easy	10 minutes	None	2

INGREDIENTS:

- 1 fennel bulb, thinly sliced
- 1 apple, thinly sliced
- 2 tablespoons chopped parsley
- 2 tablespoons olive oil
- Salt to taste

INSTRUCTIONS:

1. **In a large bowl, combine** the thinly sliced fennel and apple.
2. **Add the chopped parsley** and drizzle with olive oil.
3. **Season with salt** and toss gently to combine.
4. **Serve immediately** and enjoy a crisp, refreshing salad.

NUTRITIONAL VALUES (PER SERVING):

- Calories: 120
- Protein: 1g
- Carbohydrates: 16g
- Fat: 6g
- Fiber: 4g
- Sugar: 10g

SPINACH AND STRAWBERRY SALAD

Difficulty:	Prep Time:	Cooking Method:	Servings:
Easy	10 minutes	None	2

INGREDIENTS:

- 2 cups fresh spinach
- 1 cup sliced strawberries
- 1/4 cup crumbled feta cheese (optional)
- 2 tablespoons sliced almonds
- 2 tablespoons olive oil

INSTRUCTIONS:

1. **In a large bowl, combine** the spinach, sliced strawberries, and sliced almonds.
2. **Add the crumbled feta cheese** if using.
3. **Drizzle with olive oil** and toss gently to combine.
4. **Serve immediately** and enjoy a vibrant, nutritious salad.

NUTRITIONAL VALUES (PER SERVING):

- Calories: 180
- Protein: 5g
- Carbohydrates: 15g
- Fat: 12g
- Fiber: 4g
- Sugar: 8g

CUCUMBER SALAD

Difficulty:	Prep Time:	Cooking Method:	Servings:
Easy	10 minutes	None	2

INGREDIENTS:

- 2 cups sliced cucumber
- 2 tablespoons chopped fresh parsley
- 2 tablespoons olive oil
- Salt to taste

INSTRUCTIONS:

1. **In a large bowl, combine** the sliced cucumber and chopped parsley.
2. **Drizzle with olive oil** and season with salt.
3. **Toss gently** to combine.
4. **Serve immediately** and enjoy a refreshing, light salad.

NUTRITIONAL VALUES (PER SERVING):

- Calories: 100
- Protein: 1g
- Carbohydrates: 5g
- Fat: 9g
- Fiber: 1g
- Sugar: 2g

SOUP RECIPES

Soups are an excellent choice for soothing meals that are easy on the digestive system. Our collection of soup recipes features ingredients known for their anti-inflammatory properties and low acidity, making them ideal for managing acid reflux. These soups are not only comforting but also packed with nutrients, providing a warming and healthful option for any time of the day.

CHICKEN AND VEGETABLE SOUP

Difficulty:	Prep Time:	Cooking Method:	Servings:
Easy	15 minutes	Stovetop	2

INGREDIENTS:

- 1 chicken breast, diced
- 2 carrots, sliced
- 1 cup diced celery
- 1 cup green beans, trimmed and cut
- 1/2 cup peas
- 4 cups low-sodium chicken broth
- 1 tablespoon olive oil
- Salt and pepper to taste

INSTRUCTIONS:

1. **Heat olive oil** in a large pot over medium heat. Add the diced chicken and cook until browned.
2. **Add the carrots, celery, green beans, and peas** to the pot and cook for 5 minutes.
3. **Pour in the chicken broth** and bring to a boil. Reduce heat and simmer for 20 minutes.
4. **Season with salt and pepper** to taste.
5. **Serve hot** and enjoy a comforting, nutritious soup.

NUTRITIONAL VALUES (PER SERVING):

- Calories: 250
- Protein: 25g
- Carbohydrates: 20g
- Fat: 8g
- Fiber: 6g
- Sugar: 6g

CARROT AND GINGER SOUP

Difficulty:	Prep Time:	Cooking Method:	Servings:
Easy	**15 minutes**	**Stovetop**	**2**

INGREDIENTS:

- 4 large carrots, peeled and chopped
- 1 tablespoon grated ginger
- 4 cups low-sodium vegetable broth
- 1 tablespoon olive oil
- Salt and pepper to taste

INSTRUCTIONS:

1. **Heat olive oil** in a large pot over medium heat. Add the chopped carrots and cook until softened.
2. **Stir in the grated ginger** and cook for another minute.
3. **Pour in the vegetable broth** and bring to a boil. Reduce heat and simmer for 20 minutes.
4. **Blend the soup** using an immersion blender until smooth.
5. **Season with salt and pepper** to taste.
6. **Serve hot** and enjoy a warming, nutritious soup.

NUTRITIONAL VALUES (PER SERVING):

- Calories: 180
- Protein: 3g
- Carbohydrates: 28g
- Fat: 7g
- Fiber: 6g
- Sugar: 14g

SWEET POTATO AND BLACK BEAN SOUP

Difficulty:	Prep Time:	Cooking Method:	Servings:
Easy	**15 minutes**	**Stovetop**	**2**

INGREDIENTS:

- 2 medium sweet potatoes, peeled and cubed
- 1 can black beans, drained and rinsed
- 1 cup diced celery
- 4 cups low-sodium vegetable broth
- 1 tablespoon olive oil
- 1 teaspoon ground cumin
- Salt and pepper to taste

INSTRUCTIONS:

1. **Heat olive oil** in a large pot over medium heat. Add the diced celery and cook until softened.
2. **Add the sweet potatoes** and cook for another 5 minutes.
3. Stir in the black beans and ground cumin.
4. **Pour in the vegetable broth** and bring to a boil. Reduce heat and simmer for 20 minutes.
5. **Season with salt and pepper** to taste.
6. **Serve hot** and enjoy a hearty, flavorful soup.

NUTRITIONAL VALUES (PER SERVING):

- Calories: 300
- Protein: 10g
- Carbohydrates: 55g
- Fat: 6g
- Fiber: 14g
- Sugar: 10g

BUTTERNUT SQUASH SOUP

Difficulty:	Prep Time:	Cooking Method:	Servings:
Easy	15 minutes	Stovetop	2

INGREDIENTS:

- 1 medium butternut squash, peeled and cubed
- 1 cup diced celery
- 4 cups low-sodium vegetable broth
- 1 tablespoon olive oil
- 1/2 teaspoon ground nutmeg
- Salt and pepper to taste

INSTRUCTIONS:

1. **Heat olive oil** in a large pot over medium heat. Add the diced celery and cook until softened.
2. **Add the butternut squash** and cook for another 5 minutes.
3. **Pour in the vegetable broth** and bring to a boil. Reduce heat and simmer for 20 minutes.
4. **Blend the soup** using an immersion blender until smooth.
5. **Stir in the ground nutmeg** and season with salt and pepper.
6. **Serve hot** and enjoy a creamy, comforting soup.

NUTRITIONAL VALUES (PER SERVING):

- Calories: 200
- Protein: 3g
- Carbohydrates: 45g
- Fat: 5g
- Fiber: 10g
- Sugar: 15g

MUSHROOM AND BARLEY SOUP

Difficulty:	**Prep Time:**	**Cooking Method:**	**Servings:**
Easy	**15 minutes**	**Stovetop**	**2**

INGREDIENTS:

- 1 cup sliced mushrooms
- 1/2 cup barley
- 1 cup diced celery
- 4 cups low-sodium vegetable broth
- 1 tablespoon olive oil
- 1 teaspoon dried thyme
- Salt and pepper to taste

INSTRUCTIONS:

1. **Heat olive oil** in a large pot over medium heat. Add the diced celery and cook until softened.
2. **Add the sliced mushrooms** and cook until tender.
3. **Stir in the barley** and cook for another 2 minutes.
4. **Pour in the vegetable broth** and add the dried thyme. Bring to a boil, then reduce heat and simmer for 30 minutes.
5. **Season with salt and pepper** to taste.
6. **Serve hot** and enjoy a hearty, nutritious soup.

NUTRITIONAL VALUES (PER SERVING):

- Calories: 250
- Protein: 6g
- Carbohydrates: 45g
- Fat: 6g
- Fiber: 8g
- Sugar: 6g

FENNEL AND LEEK SOUP

Difficulty:	Prep Time:	Cooking Method:	Servings:
Easy	**15 minutes**	**Stovetop**	**2**

INGREDIENTS:

- 2 cups sliced fennel
- 1 cup sliced leeks (white and light green parts only)
- 4 cups low-sodium vegetable broth
- 1 tablespoon olive oil
- 1 teaspoon dried thyme
- Salt and pepper to taste

INSTRUCTIONS:

1. Heat olive oil in a large pot over medium heat. Add the sliced fennel and leeks, and cook until softened.
2. **Stir in the dried thyme** and cook for another minute.
3. **Pour in the vegetable broth** and bring to a boil. Reduce heat and simmer for 20 minutes.
4. **Season with salt and pepper** to taste.
5. **Serve hot** and enjoy a soothing, flavorful soup.

NUTRITIONAL VALUES (PER SERVING):

- Calories: 180
- Protein: 3g
- Carbohydrates: 28g
- Fat: 7g
- Fiber: 6g
- Sugar: 14g

ZUCCHINI AND BASIL SOUP

Difficulty:	**Prep Time:**	**Cooking Method:**	**Servings:**
Easy	15 minutes	Stovetop	2

INGREDIENTS:

- 2 medium zucchinis, chopped
- 1 cup fresh basil leaves
- 4 cups low-sodium vegetable broth
- 1 tablespoon olive oil
- Salt and pepper to taste

INSTRUCTIONS:

1. **Heat olive oil** in a large pot over medium heat. Add the chopped zucchini and cook until softened.
2. **Stir in the fresh basil leaves** and cook for another minute.
3. **Pour in the vegetable broth** and bring to a boil. Reduce heat and simmer for 20 minutes.
4. **Blend the soup** using an immersion blender until smooth.
5. **Season with salt and pepper** to taste.
6. **Serve hot** and enjoy a fresh, nutritious soup.

NUTRITIONAL VALUES (PER SERVING):

- Calories: 160
- Protein: 4g
- Carbohydrates: 18g
- Fat: 8g
- Fiber: 4g
- Sugar: 8g

CAULIFLOWER AND PARSNIP SOUP

Difficulty:	Prep Time:	Cooking Method:	Servings:
Easy	**15 minutes**	**Stovetop**	**2**

INGREDIENTS:

- 1 small cauliflower, chopped
- 2 parsnips, peeled and chopped
- 4 cups low-sodium vegetable broth
- 1 tablespoon olive oil
- 1 teaspoon ground nutmeg
- Salt and pepper to taste

INSTRUCTIONS:

1. **Heat olive oil** in a large pot over medium heat. Add the chopped cauliflower and parsnips, and cook until softened.
2. **Stir in the ground nutmeg** and cook for another minute.
3. **Pour in the vegetable broth** and bring to a boil. Reduce heat and simmer for 20 minutes.
4. **Blend the soup** using an immersion blender until smooth.
5. **Season with salt and pepper** to taste.
6. **Serve hot** and enjoy a creamy, comforting soup.

NUTRITIONAL VALUES (PER SERVING):

- Calories: 180
- Protein: 4g
- Carbohydrates: 28g
- Fat: 7g
- Fiber: 6g
- Sugar: 10g

GREEN PEA SOUP

Difficulty:	Prep Time:	Cooking Method:	Servings:
Easy	**10 minutes**	**Stovetop**	**2**

INGREDIENTS:

- 2 cups green peas (fresh or frozen)
- 1/4 cup fresh parsley leaves
- 4 cups low-sodium vegetable broth
- 1 tablespoon olive oil
- Salt and pepper to taste

INSTRUCTIONS:

1. **Heat olive oil** in a large pot over medium heat. Add the green peas and cook until heated through.
2. **Stir in the fresh parsley leaves** and cook for another minute.
3. **Pour in the vegetable broth** and bring to a boil. Reduce heat and simmer for 10 minutes.
4. **Blend the soup** using an immersion blender until smooth.
5. **Season with salt and pepper** to taste.
6. **Serve hot** and enjoy a refreshing, nutritious soup.

NUTRITIONAL VALUES (PER SERVING):

- Calories: 160
- Protein: 6g
- Carbohydrates: 24g
- Fat: 6g
- Fiber: 8g
- Sugar: 10g

KALE AND WHITE BEAN SOUP

Difficulty:	**Prep Time:**	**Cooking Method:**	**Servings:**
Easy	**15 minutes**	**Stovetop**	**2**

INGREDIENTS:

- 2 cups chopped kale
- 1 can white beans, drained and rinsed
- 1 cup diced celery
- 4 cups low-sodium vegetable broth
- 1 tablespoon olive oil
- 1 teaspoon dried thyme
- Salt and pepper to taste

INSTRUCTIONS:

1. **Heat olive oil** in a large pot over medium heat. Add the diced celery and cook until softened.
2. **Add the chopped kale and white beans** and cook for another 5 minutes.
3. **Stir in the dried thyme.**
4. **Pour in the vegetable broth** and bring to a boil. Reduce heat and simmer for 20 minutes.
5. **Season with salt and pepper** to taste.
6. **Serve hot** and enjoy a hearty, nutritious soup.

NUTRITIONAL VALUES (PER SERVING):

- Calories: 220
- Protein: 12g
- Carbohydrates: 30g
- Fat: 8g
- Fiber: 10g
- Sugar: 4g

HORS D'OEUVRES AND SNACKS

Finding the right snacks and hors d'oeuvres can be challenging when managing acid reflux, but our selection offers delicious solutions that are both satisfying and reflux-friendly. Each recipe is designed to provide a burst of flavor without triggering symptoms, using ingredients that support digestive health and keep you feeling full and happy between meals.

CUCUMBER AND HUMMUS BITES

Difficulty:	Prep Time:	Cooking Method:	Servings:
Easy	10 minutes	None	2

INGREDIENTS:

- 1 cucumber, sliced into rounds
- 1/2 cup hummus
- Fresh parsley for garnish

INSTRUCTIONS:

1. **Slice the cucumber** into thick rounds.
2. **Spoon a dollop of hummus** onto each cucumber slice.
3. **Garnish with a sprig of parsley.**
4. **Serve immediately** and enjoy a refreshing, healthy snack.

NUTRITIONAL VALUES (PER SERVING):

- Calories: 120
- Protein: 4g
- Carbohydrates: 16g
- Fat: 5g
- Fiber: 4g
- Sugar: 2g

AVOCADO DEVILED EGGS

Difficulty:	Prep Time:	Cooking Method:	Servings:
Easy	**15 minutes**	**Boiling**	**2**

INGREDIENTS:

- 4 hard-boiled eggs, halved
- 1 avocado, mashed
- 1 tablespoon Greek yogurt (low-fat)
- Salt and pepper to taste
- Fresh chives for garnish

INSTRUCTIONS:

1. **Boil the eggs**, peel them, and cut in half lengthwise. Remove yolks.
2. **Mash the avocado** with the Greek yogurt.
3. **Season with salt and pepper.**
4. **Spoon the mixture** back into the egg whites.
5. **Garnish with fresh chives** and serve immediately.

NUTRITIONAL VALUES (PER SERVING):

- Calories: 160
- Protein: 12g
- Carbohydrates: 6g
- Fat: 10g
- Fiber: 4g
- Sugar: 1g

BAKED SWEET POTATO FRIES

Difficulty:	Prep Time:	Cooking Method:	Servings:
Easy	10 minutes	Baking	2

INGREDIENTS:

- 2 medium sweet potatoes, peeled and cut into fries
- 2 tablespoons olive oil
- 1 teaspoon smoked paprika (optional)
- Salt and pepper to taste

INSTRUCTIONS:

1. **Preheat the oven** to 425°F (220°C).
2. **Toss the sweet potato fries** with olive oil, smoked paprika, salt, and pepper.
3. **Spread in a single layer** on a baking sheet.
4. **Bake for 20-25 minutes**, flipping halfway through, until crispy.
5. **Serve hot** and enjoy a healthy snack.

NUTRITIONAL VALUES (PER SERVING):

- Calories: 200
- Protein: 2g
- Carbohydrates: 34g
- Fat: 7g
- Fiber: 5g
- Sugar: 7g

TURKEY AND CUCUMBER ROLL-UPS

Difficulty:	Prep Time:	Cooking Method:	Servings:
Easy	**10 minutes**	**None**	**2**

INGREDIENTS:

- 4 slices of turkey breast
- 1 cucumber, sliced into thin strips
- 1/4 cup hummus
- Fresh dill for garnish

INSTRUCTIONS:

1. **Lay out the turkey slices flat**.
2. **Spread a thin layer of hummus** on each slice.
3. **Place cucumber strips** on top of the hummus.
4. **Roll up the turkey slices** and secure with a toothpick if needed.
5. **Garnish with fresh dill** and serve immediately.

NUTRITIONAL VALUES (PER SERVING):

- Calories: 150
- Protein: 15g
- Carbohydrates: 8g
- Fat: 6g
- Fiber: 2g
- Sugar: 2g

ZUCCHINI CHIPS

Difficulty:	Prep Time:	Cooking Method:	Servings:
Easy	10 minutes	Baking	2

INGREDIENTS:

- 2 zucchinis, thinly sliced
- 2 tablespoons olive oil
- 1 teaspoon dried oregano
- Salt and pepper to taste

INSTRUCTIONS:

1. **Preheat the oven** to 225°F (110°C).
2. **Toss the zucchini slices** with olive oil, dried oregano, salt, and pepper.
3. **Arrange in a single layer** on a baking sheet lined with parchment paper.
4. **Bake for 1-2 hours**, until crispy, flipping halfway through.
5. **Serve immediately** and enjoy a crunchy, healthy snack.

NUTRITIONAL VALUES (PER SERVING):

- Calories: 100
- Protein: 2g
- Carbohydrates: 8g
- Fat: 7g
- Fiber: 2g
- Sugar: 4g

CARROT AND CELERY STICKS WITH YOGURT DIP

Difficulty:	Prep Time:	Cooking Method:	Servings:
Easy	**10 minutes**	**None**	**2**

INGREDIENTS:

- 2 large carrots, peeled and cut into sticks
- 2 celery stalks, cut into sticks
- 1/2 cup low-fat Greek yogurt
- 1 teaspoon dried dill
- Salt and pepper to taste

INSTRUCTIONS:

1. **Peel and cut the carrots** and celery into sticks.
2. **In a small bowl**, combine the Greek yogurt, dried dill, salt, and pepper.
3. **Serve the carrot and celery sticks** with the yogurt dip.
4. **Enjoy a crunchy, healthy snack.**

NUTRITIONAL VALUES (PER SERVING):

- Calories: 100
- Protein: 5g
- Carbohydrates: 12g
- Fat: 4g
- Fiber: 3g
- Sugar: 6g

RICE CAKES WITH AVOCADO SPREAD

Difficulty:	**Prep Time:**	**Cooking Method:**	**Servings:**
Easy	**10 minutes**	**None**	**2**

INGREDIENTS:

- 4 plain rice cakes
- 1 avocado, mashed
- 1 teaspoon olive oil
- Salt and pepper to taste
- Fresh parsley for garnish

INSTRUCTIONS:

1. **Mash the avocado** with olive oil, salt, and pepper.
2. **Spread the avocado mixture** onto the rice cakes.
3. **Garnish with fresh parsley.**
4. **Serve immediately** and enjoy a light, nutritious snack.

NUTRITIONAL VALUES (PER SERVING):

- Calories: 150
- Protein: 2g
- Carbohydrates: 20g
- Fat: 8g
- Fiber: 5g
- Sugar: 1g

APPLE SLICES WITH ALMOND BUTTER

Difficulty:	**Prep Time:**	**Cooking Method:**	**Servings:**
Easy	5 minutes	None	2

INGREDIENTS:

- 2 apples, sliced
- 1/4 cup almond butter

INSTRUCTIONS:

1. Slice the apples into wedges.
2. Serve the apple slices with almond butter for dipping.
3. Enjoy a sweet and satisfying snack.

NUTRITIONAL VALUES (PER SERVING):

- Calories: 220
- Protein: 4g
- Carbohydrates: 32g
- Fat: 10g
- Fiber: 6g
- Sugar: 20g

CRISPY KALE CHIPS

Difficulty:	Prep Time:	Cooking Method:	Servings:
Easy	10 minutes	Baking	2

INGREDIENTS:

- 1 bunch kale, washed and torn into pieces
- 2 tablespoons olive oil
- 1 teaspoon smoked paprika (optional)
- Salt to taste

INSTRUCTIONS:

1. **Preheat the oven** to 300°F (150°C).
2. **Toss the kale pieces** with olive oil, smoked paprika, and salt.
3. **Arrange in a single layer** on a baking sheet.
4. **Bake for 20-25 minutes**, until crispy.
5. **Serve immediately** and enjoy a healthy, crunchy snack.

NUTRITIONAL VALUES (PER SERVING):

- Calories: 100
- Protein: 2g
- Carbohydrates: 8g
- Fat: 7g
- Fiber: 2g
- Sugar: 1g

CHICKPEA AND AVOCADO MASH ON WHOLE GRAIN TOAST

Difficulty:	Prep Time:	Cooking Method:	Servings:
Easy	10 minutes	None	2

INGREDIENTS:

- 1 can chickpeas, drained and rinsed
- 1 avocado, mashed
- 4 slices whole grain bread
- 1 teaspoon olive oil
- Salt and pepper to taste

INSTRUCTIONS:

1. **Mash the chickpeas** with the avocado and olive oil.
2. **Season with salt and pepper.**
3. Spread the chickpea and avocado mash onto the whole grain toast.
4. **Serve immediately** and enjoy a nutritious, satisfying snack.

NUTRITIONAL VALUES (PER SERVING):

- Calories: 250
- Protein: 8g
- Carbohydrates: 32g
- Fat: 10g
- Fiber: 10g
- Sugar: 2g

DESSERTS

Enjoying desserts without the worry of acid reflux is possible with our carefully curated recipes. These desserts are made with ingredients that are low in acidity and gentle on the stomach, allowing you to indulge your sweet tooth without discomfort. Each recipe provides a delightful treat that balances taste and health, ensuring you can enjoy dessert time while maintaining your digestive wellness.

BAKED APPLES WITH HONEY AND WALNUTS

Difficulty:	Prep Time:	Cooking Method:	Servings:
Easy	10 minutes	Baking	2

INGREDIENTS:

- 2 apples, cored and sliced
- 1 tablespoon honey
- 2 tablespoons chopped walnuts

INSTRUCTIONS:

1. **Preheat the oven** to 350°F (175°C).
2. **Arrange the apple slices** in a baking dish.
3. **Drizzle with honey** and sprinkle with chopped walnuts.
4. **Bake for 20-25 minutes** until the apples are tender.
5. **Serve warm** and enjoy a sweet, comforting dessert.

NUTRITIONAL VALUES (PER SERVING):

- Calories: 180
- Protein: 2g
- Carbohydrates: 36g
- Fat: 5g
- Fiber: 4g
- Sugar: 28g

BANANA OAT COOKIES

Difficulty:	Prep Time:	Cooking Method:	Servings:
Easy	10 minutes	Baking	2

INGREDIENTS:

- 2 ripe bananas, mashed
- 1 cup rolled oats
- 1/4 cup raisins
- 1 teaspoon vanilla extract

INSTRUCTIONS:

1. **Preheat the oven** to 350°F (175°C).
2. **In a bowl, combine** the mashed bananas, rolled oats, raisins, and vanilla extract.
3. **Drop spoonfuls of the mixture** onto a baking sheet lined with parchment paper.
4. **Bake for 15-20 minutes** until golden brown.
5. **Let cool** and enjoy a healthy, chewy cookie.

NUTRITIONAL VALUES (PER SERVING):

- Calories: 150
- Protein: 3g
- Carbohydrates: 33g
- Fat: 2g
- Fiber: 4g
- Sugar: 14g

BANANA RICE PUDDING

Difficulty:	Prep Time:	Cooking Method:	Servings:
Easy	10 minutes	Stovetop	2

INGREDIENTS:

- 1 cup cooked white rice
- 1 cup hemp milk
- 1 ripe, non-acidic banana (such as the Burro or Manzano variety), mashed
- 1 tablespoon agave syrup
- 1/2 teaspoon vanilla extract
- 1/4 teaspoon ground cinnamon

INSTRUCTIONS:

1. **In a medium saucepan**, combine the cooked rice and hemp milk over medium heat.
2. **Stir in the mashed banana**, agave syrup, vanilla extract, and ground cinnamon.
3. **Cook, stirring frequently**, until the mixture thickens and becomes creamy, about 10 minutes.
4. **Remove from heat** and let it cool slightly.
5. **Serve warm or chilled**, as desired. Enjoy a comforting and acid-reflux friendly dessert.

NUTRITIONAL VALUES (PER SERVING):

- Calories: 200
- Protein: 4g
- Carbohydrates: 40g
- Fat: 3g
- Fiber: 2g
- Sugar: 10g

MANGO SMOOTHIE

Difficulty:	Prep Time:	Cooking Method:	Servings:
Easy	**5 minutes**	**Blending**	**2**

INGREDIENTS:

- 1 ripe mango, peeled and chopped
- 1/2 cup hemp milk
- 1/2 cup Greek yogurt (low-fat)
- 1 tablespoon honey
- Ice cubes

INSTRUCTIONS:

1. **In a blender, combine** the mango, hemp milk, Greek yogurt, honey, and ice cubes.
2. **Blend until smooth** and creamy.
3. **Pour into glasses** and serve immediately.
4. **Enjoy a refreshing,** tropical dessert.

NUTRITIONAL VALUES (PER SERVING):

- Calories: 220
- Protein: 6g
- Carbohydrates: 36g
- Fat: 8g
- Fiber: 4g
- Sugar: 30g

STRAWBERRY ALMOND PARFAIT

Difficulty:	**Prep Time:**	**Cooking Method:**	**Servings:**
Easy	**10 minutes**	**None**	**2**

INGREDIENTS:

- 1 cup Greek yogurt (low-fat)
- 1/2 cup fresh strawberries
- 1/4 cup granola (low-sugar)
- 2 tablespoons sliced almonds
- 1 tablespoon honey

INSTRUCTIONS:

1. **In two serving glasses,** layer Greek yogurt, fresh strawberries, granola, and sliced almonds.
2. **Drizzle with honey.**
3. **Serve immediately and enjoy** a delightful, layered dessert.

NUTRITIONAL VALUES (PER SERVING):

- Calories: 200
- Protein: 8g
- Carbohydrates: 28g
- Fat: 7g
- Fiber: 4g
- Sugar: 18g

PUMPKIN CUSTARD

Difficulty:	Prep Time:	Cooking Method:	Servings:
Easy	10 minutes	Baking	2

INGREDIENTS:

- 1 cup pumpkin puree
- 1/2 cup low-fat Greek yogurt
- 2 tablespoons honey
- 1 teaspoon vanilla extract
- 1/2 teaspoon ground ginger
- 1/4 teaspoon ground cloves
- 1/4 teaspoon ground nutmeg (optional)

INSTRUCTIONS:

1. **Preheat the oven** to 350°F (175°C).
2. **In a bowl, mix** the pumpkin puree, Greek yogurt, honey, vanilla extract, ground ginger, and ground cloves.
3. **In a bowl, mix** the pumpkin puree, Greek yogurt, honey, vanilla extract, ground ginger, and ground cloves.
4. **Pour the mixture** into two custard cups.
5. **Bake for 20-25 minutes**, until set.
6. **Serve warm or chilled** and enjoy a creamy, spiced dessert.

NUTRITIONAL VALUES (PER SERVING):

- Calories: 180
- Protein: 8g
- Carbohydrates: 32g
- Fat: 2g
- Fiber: 4g
- Sugar: 24g

OATMEAL RAISIN COOKIES

Difficulty:	Prep Time:	Cooking Method:	Servings:
Easy	10 minutes	Baking	2

INGREDIENTS:

- 1 cup rolled oats
- 1/2 cup mashed bananas
- 1/4 cup raisins
- 1 teaspoon vanilla extract
- 1/2 teaspoon ground cinnamon (if tolerated)

INSTRUCTIONS:

1. **Preheat the oven** to 350°F (175°C).
2. **In a bowl, combine** the rolled oats, mashed bananas, raisins, vanilla extract, and ground cinnamon (if using).
3. **Drop spoonfuls of the mixture** onto a baking sheet lined with parchment paper.
4. **Bake for 15-20 minutes**, until golden brown.
5. **Let cool** and enjoy a healthy, chewy cookie.

NUTRITIONAL VALUES (PER SERVING):

- Calories: 150
- Protein: 3g
- Carbohydrates: 33g
- Fat: 2g
- Fiber: 4g
- Sugar: 14g

PEACH AND RASPBERRY SORBET

Difficulty:	Prep Time:	Cooking Method:	Servings:
Easy	10 minutes (plus freezing time)	Freezing	2

INGREDIENTS:

- 2 ripe peaches, peeled and chopped
- 1/2 cup fresh raspberries
- 2 tablespoons honey
- 1/4 cup water

INSTRUCTIONS:

1. In a blender, combine the peaches, raspberries, honey, and water.
2. Blend until smooth.
3. Pour the mixture into a shallow dish and freeze for 2-3 hours, stirring every 30 minutes.
4. Scoop into bowls and serve immediately.
5. Enjoy a refreshing, fruity sorbet.

NUTRITIONAL VALUES (PER SERVING):

- Calories: 100
- Protein: 1g
- Carbohydrates: 26g
- Fat: 0g
- Fiber: 4g
- Sugar: 22g

CARROT CAKE BITES

Difficulty:	Prep Time:	Cooking Method:	Servings:
Easy	**15 minutes**	**None**	**2**

INGREDIENTS:

- 1 cup grated carrots
- 1/2 cup rolled oats
- 1/4 cup raisins
- 2 tablespoons almond butter
- 1 tablespoon honey
- 1 teaspoon vanilla extract

INSTRUCTIONS:

1. **In a bowl**, combine the grated carrots, rolled oats, raisins, almond butter, honey, and vanilla extract.
2. **Mix well until combined.**
3. **Form into bite-sized balls** and place on a baking sheet.
4. **Refrigerate for 1 hour to set.**
5. **Serve chilled and enjoy** a sweet, nutritious snack.

NUTRITIONAL VALUES (PER SERVING):

- Calories: 180
- Protein: 4g
- Carbohydrates: 32g
- Fat: 6g
- Fiber: 4g
- Sugar: 18g

QUINOA PUDDING

Difficulty:	**Prep Time:**	**Cooking Method:**	**Servings:**
Easy	10 minutes	Stovetop	2

INGREDIENTS:

- 1/2 cup quinoa, rinsed
- 1 cup hemp milk
- 1 tablespoon honey
- 1 teaspoon vanilla extract
- Fresh berries for topping

INSTRUCTIONS:

1. **In a saucepan**, combine the quinoa and almond milk.
2. **Bring to a boil**, then reduce heat and simmer for 15-20 minutes, until the quinoa is tender and the milk is absorbed.
3. **Stir in the honey and vanilla extract.**
4. **Serve warm or chilled**, topped with fresh berries.
5. **Enjoy** a creamy, nutritious dessert.

NUTRITIONAL VALUES (PER SERVING):

- Calories: 220
- Protein: 6g
- Carbohydrates: 38g
- Fat: 6g
- Fiber: 4g
- Sugar: 12g

Through our array of recipes, we hope you have discovered the joy and ease of preparing meals that support your digestive health. With each meal, you are taking proactive steps toward better health and a more comfortable lifestyle.

MEASUREMENT UNIT CONVERSION TABLE

Accurate measurements are crucial for successful cooking, particularly when managing a condition like acid reflux where specific ingredients and quantities are key to avoiding symptoms. This measurement conversion table is designed to assist you in seamlessly transitioning between different units of measurement commonly found in recipes. Whether you're converting volume, weight, or temperature, this table ensures that you have the precise information needed to follow recipes correctly and make adjustments as necessary.

VOLUME CONVERSION

US Volume	Metric Volume	Equivalents
1 teaspoon (tsp)	5 milliliters (ml)	-
1 tablespoon (tbsp)	15 milliliters (ml)	3 teaspoons
1 fluid ounce (fl oz)	30 milliliters (ml)	2 tablespoons
1 cup (c)	240 milliliters (ml)	8 fluid ounces
1 pint (pt)	480 milliliters (ml)	2 cups, 16 fluid ounces
1 quart (qt)	960 milliliters (ml)	2 pints, 4 cups, 32 fluid ounces
1 gallon (gal)	3.8 liters (L)	4 quarts, 8 pints, 16 cups, 128 fluid ounces

WEIGHT CONVERSION

US Weight	Metric Weight	Equivalents
1 ounce (oz)	28 grams (g)	-
1 pound (lb)	454 grams (g)	16 ounces
1 pound (lb)	0.45 kilograms (kg)	16 ounces

TEMPERATURE CONVERSIONS

Fahrenheit (°F)	Celsius (°C)
32°F	0°C
100°F	37.8°C
212°F	100°C
350°F	177°C
375°F	190°C
400°F	204°C
425°F	218°C
450°F	232°C

BONUS

Thank You for Choosing "The Complete Acid Reflux Diet Cookbook"!

Your commitment to improving your health and managing acid reflux shows just how much you care about your well-being. I am truly honored that you have decided to embark on this journey with me.

As a token of my appreciation, I am excited to offer you 3 exclusive bonuses for free:

- **60-Day Meal Plan**: A structured, easy-to-follow plan designed to improve your health and reduce reflux symptoms.
- **Lifestyle Adjustments to Improve Acid Reflux**: Practical tips to adjust your lifestyle and see real results.
- **Natural Remedies and Management**: Discover the best natural solutions to manage and alleviate acid reflux.

To receive these bonuses, simply send an email to: <u>nicoleeverglen@gmail</u>.com and you'll get the material delivered right to your inbox.

Your opinion means the world to me. I invite you to share an honest review on Amazon. Your feedback will help others discover this book and find relief from acid reflux.

Thank you again for allowing me to be a part of your journey to better health. Together we can make a difference.

With deep gratitude,

Nicòle Everglen

CONCLUSION

As we reach the end of this book, let's take a moment to reflect on knowledge we've shared towards managing acid reflux. Our exploration began with a thorough understanding of the science behind acid reflux, providing insights into the mechanisms of the condition, its symptoms, and the distinction between GERD and LPR. We leaned into the causes and risk factors, highlighting the importance of recognizing when medical consultation or even surgical intervention might be necessary.

In the second chapter, we focused on diet and nutrition, emphasizing the critical role they play in managing acid reflux. We identified a comprehensive list of allowed and prohibited foods, providing clear guidance on what to include and avoid in your diet. This chapter served as a valuable resource, equipping you with the nutritional knowledge to execute a dietary reform.

The final chapter offered a diverse array of recipes, from hearty breakfasts to delectable desserts, all designed to be gentle on the digestive system while being flavorful and satisfying. These recipes, crafted with care and consideration, aimed to make your culinary journey enjoyable and supportive of your health goals.

Looking back, in a short time this book has provided you with a well-rounded understanding of acid reflux, the importance of diet in managing the condition, and practical, delicious recipes to incorporate into your daily life. Our final advice for you is simple: Managing acid reflux is a continuous effort that requires awareness, dedication, and informed choices; stay committed to your health, listen to your body, and enjoy the process of nourishing yourself with foods that support your well-being.

Made in the USA
Las Vegas, NV
20 November 2024

12196844R00059